POLES APART

By Michelle McMeekin

Michelle McMeekin

Published by
Chipmunkapublishing
PO Box 6872
Brentwood
Essex CM13 1ZT
United Kingdom

http://www.chipmunkapublishing.com

Edited by Folake Akinbode

POLES APART

"THERE IS NO HEALTH WITHOUT MENTAL HEALTH"

Today I have come a long, long way and finally decided to put pen to paper and tell my story of my descent into the hell of serious mental health. How I have dealt with stigma, lost my identity, nearly my life and the long, long climb back to sanity and an understanding of my condition. I suffer from Bi-polar disorder (Manic Depression) and although it will never be my friend, I have learnt to accept that it is a part of me and I think it has made me a stronger, better and more understanding person.

Michelle McMeekin

POLES APART

Acknowledgements

Firstly I would like to thank my dear Mum and Dad, who have been there from the very beginning.
My Billy, my rock who was there for me from the last breakdown. The only man I have ever known who truly loves me for just being me. My wonderful brother 'Stu',
"True friends" – they know who they are.

Kristy and Lauren – My angels sent from God as a reminder that life isn't easy but after tremendous hardship there can be great joy. They have been my saviours.

Last, but not least, my wonderful Nanna (departed) who still stands by my side.

Michelle McMeekin

POLES APART

I decided to write my story not because I want pity, or not even for people to say hasn't she done well overcoming her problems, but in the hope and belief that if one person who is currently experiencing the sheer hell I have gone through many times in the past, can pick up this book and I can give them a glimmer of hope at the end of the black, black tunnel I will truly have achieved something.

If you have ever suffered from serious mental health problems you will never have the same outlook on life again. I changed at 17 when I had my first experience and I have continued changing until I have finally become my true self (20 years later).

I could have become bitter but that is a wasted emotion. I have become more spiritual and looked at things in the bigger picture.

Up until 10 years ago I think I believed in God. I didn't hold with the theory that when you are dead that's it but I never really gave much thought to the spiritual part of my life. I only went to church for weddings, christenings and funerals. Today I personally believe there is something else. Although I don't want to die as I love my children, husband and family so much I am not scared of death. This is only my belief and you will see how I have come to this conclusion when you read my story.

Everybody has turning points in their lives when their life goes in a different direction. I can pinpoint the day when I decided to write my book and help other sufferers by becoming a volunteer at MIND. I had toyed with the idea of writing a book before but something happened to me that day that had a profound effect of me. I was reading an article in the paper and the article was about Achievement Awards for People. It might have been the Daily Mirror's "Pride of Britain". I'm not sure but that doesn't matter as it was the contents of the article that had an effect on me. It was the true story of a husband and wife who were both professionals. They had worked hard in their careers, had a nice lifestyle and plenty of money. They wanted a baby but couldn't conceive naturally. They had IVF. I'm not sure how many courses of IVF they had but eventually they had a baby – a precious baby. But the wife got serious post-natal depression. Now the difference between having serious post-natal depression and normal post-natal depression is the difference between having pneumonia and a cold. She became very ill and their lives were turned upside down. The husband had no experience of dealing with mental health problems and he struggled to cope. One day when the baby was about 4 months old she went off in her car and threw herself of beachhead cliffs. The husband now patrols the cliffs and has saved countless lives by persuading people not to throw themselves off. Even whilst I am writing this I have had to break off twice to cry as it has had such an effect on me. I would like to meet this man one day. The thing is that poor, poor dead lady could have been me and I understand exactly what she was going through. People who have never suffered with <u>serious</u> mental health problems and it has to be serious (I am not deriding any other forms of mental health, only when it is serious you become psychotic (mad)). Years ago you would have been put in a straight jacket and locked away in a Mental Institution. People will say how she could leave her baby and husband, she couldn't have loved them. That is utter rubbish. She would have been so ill and out of touch with reality she wouldn't have known what she was doing.

Other factors have made me put pen to paper as well. I believe my Nanna who sadly took her own life after a very hard and serious depression is guiding me and wanting me to help others now I am strong and well myself. The day after reading the above article I rang MIND to see about volunteering work. I had a chat with a very nice lady called Alison who is in charge of volunteers at Darlington MIND. She seemed very pleased I wanted to be a volunteer. I came off the phone and immediately went to my car as I was due somewhere. As I turned the ignition, the radio, which had been missing for weeks, fell out of the sun visor. I put it on and there was a programme on Radio 2 discussing a lady lawyer in the USA who had killed herself by jumping from a tower block. A listener had just said she was selfish and discussion commenced. Another listener said no-one could judge unless they had suffered from mental health problems (if you are depressed you are seriously unhappy, if you are seriously depressed you are dead inside).   Someone who has suffered would never judge. I only feel deep, deep sorrow that another soul has been in such torment with no help and a life wasted. I knew then that I had to do something (it was like a calling!). There are so many people out there too ill to speak for themselves.

My father had a breakdown when he was 22 but thankfully he got better and wasn't ill again only now and again things would get on top of him. He always worked and never took any medication. When I was about 11 I asked my Mum "What's wrong with Dad?" "He's suffering with his nerves but he'll be fine it's nothing for you to worry about" she said "What are nerves Mum?" I said "It's hard to understand love and hopefully you'll never find out" she said. These words would haunt me.

I was always a worrier as a child. We lived in a semi with open plan stairs from the living room to the landing. My bedroom was nearest to the top of the stairs. My parents are wonderful and they tried their best when I was a child but they always struggled with money. Poor dad always had to do overtime at work.   If I heard them discussing money problems I would lie awake and worry. I don't think Stuart my younger and only brother was ever really aware but I was much more

POLES APART

sensitive (an old head on young shoulders). I never wanted to bother Mum and Dad with my worries so my beloved Nanna was my confidante. She was wonderful my Nanna. She was so kind, thoughtful and always willing to put others before herself. She had my Uncle Paul when she was going through the change of life and consequently he was born with fluid on the brain and other complications. When he was 5 he was hit on the head with a hammer by a playmate and he went blind. My Nanna dedicated her life to the taking care of him. Most of her family i.e. my Granddad and Uncle Keith were selfish and did little to help her but she didn't moan she just got on with it. Even as a small child I had a close bond with her and I thought she was amazing. When I was about 13 I entered a competition with a local taxi firm. You had to write an essay on someone who inspired you. I wrote about my Nanna. I was one of the winners and Nana got to enjoy an all expenses paid day out to the seaside. In the later stages of her life she was crippled with arthritis but she never complained. When I was 14 and Stuart 12 she decided she wanted to go on holiday with us. She gave me the money and I looked us on a mini-break to Paris. We had a lovely time. When we came home Nanna told Mum and Dad how proud of me she was. I had organised the whole holiday and because I was doing French at school we had got by. She was getting very frail and helpless and relied on me and Stu on holiday. I was glowing with her praise.

She had been a tower of strength but when my Uncle Paul reached 30 (she had been told he would live only until he was about 10) she was 70 years old, her body couldn't cope anymore. Uncle Paul had to go into a home. Nanna was devastated. Granddad died of lung cancer and the following year Uncle Paul died. Nanna sunk into a deep depression from which she never recovered. At this stage in my life I was suffering with my first breakdown and as I was very ill myself I couldn't help her. Even when I became better I didn't spend that much time with her. As I have said previously, up until I was 16 I loved to be with her. She was still very ill and not the Nanna I knew, and in my ignorance I felt if I spent long periods of time with her I would become ill again. She hung herself when I was 20 and for a long time a part of me felt guilty that I hadn't been there for her. I know now in my heart that she doesn't blame me as she knew I was getting over being ill. I still feel close to her and believe she is my Guardian Angel watching over me.

My Mum was a barmaid and although she was a lovely Mum she had little confidence in her abilities but my Dad, who was a Centre laid Turner in a factory was quite intelligent. He said his biggest regret was that he hadn't stuck in at school and he had ended up in a hard low paid job. Because I was bright at school they encouraged me to do well and I would have a better life. As a child you don't know you own mind and I believed that if I did well at school, got

POLES APART

a good job and lots of money my life would be just perfect with no worries. So from the age of 11 when I started Long field Comprehensive School I was the perfect student. I wasn't what you would call a natural, I was a Trier. I was in the top half of the top two classes (there was a tier system in place at Long field; 2 top classes, 3 averages and 1 bottom). For 5 years at Long field I worried constantly about not passing my exams, being unable to get a job, becoming a failure and letting everyone down. It didn't help that I was a teenager in the 1980s – it was doom and glom everywhere. Margaret Thatcher's diabolical government, unemployment at 3.5 million. Even the teachers put the pressure on. You had to stick in as there was so much competition for so few jobs. My teachers all believed that I would go to the sixth form college and do my 'A' levels so even my options weren't the ones I wanted to do. I wanted to learn to type but I had to do french. I was going to be an academic they thought not a typist. But something told me I'd had enough. Every night I did roughly 2 hours homework and I new college would push me over the edge. I left school with 5 'O' levels and on the day in June when I left I felt like a great big weight had been lifted from my shoulders. I had got a place on an YTS training scheme at Darlington Borough Council and I was due to start in the September. I had been working in Fine Fare Supermarket on a Saturday whilst still at school so I increased my hours over the summer. Looking back this is one of the happiest times in my life. Without any of the worries of school weighing me down I became more happy and carefree and felt my life had just begun and after working so hard at school I thought I would get my just reward. How naïve I was!

I truly believed in those days that you made you own luck and if you worked hard you got rewarded. I still believe this theory to a degree but if you have mental or physical health problems you aren't in control of your life. You could be the best high flying lawyer in the world but if you have a breakdown your life will coming crashing down around your ears. You can loose everything. Friends (only true friends will stick by you) others will treat you like you have the plague. Your job if you can't recover from the breakdown. So then you have financial worries and, in theory, if you had no supportive family to fall back on, you could be out on the streets. The NHS is hopeless in dealing with Mental Health. Only a very small percentage of the overall budget goes on Mental Health. If you've ever had to stay in a NHS mental hospital you will know what I am talking about. They are like hell on earth. The NHS can only cope with crisis situations.

So if you go to your doctor (I would at this point say that since my third breakdown and when I was diagnosed with Bi-polar, Dr. Young my doctor, has been very good with me and I would like to thank her for all her help and support) feeling stressed or depressed and unable to cope invariably they will give you anti-depressants and you will wait for months to see a physiatrist. By then you could be very seriously mentally ill and suicidal.

One in four people are supposed to suffer from mental health problems at some point in their lives. But there still isn't enough money put into this aspect of the NHS. Although undoubtedly things are a bit better than they were say 50 years ago, there is still stigma attached. If someone has a serious physical illness i.e. cancer, nobody in their right mind would dream of saying "well they look all right to me". But you could be in the grips of psychosis (madness people with Manic Depression or Schizophrenia get when really ill) and some people would say "pull yourself together". Or "I saw him/her in town and they didn't look ill!" Personally, I think that this is one of the hardest things to cope with. You don't look ill, so some cruel, insensitive people don't think you are ill at all.

When I started at the Town Hall in the September I was 16. I worked for 3 months in the Environmental Health Department which I liked very much. You weren't under any pressure just learning the way things were done at a gentle pace. I also attended college one day a week on a day release basis doing a BTEC National Course in Business Studies (everybody on the Council YTS had to have at least 4 'O' levels and agree to go to college to be on the YTS. Things were fine until I left Environmental Health at

Christmas. I had to do an outside placement for 3 months. I was given a placement at Reg Vardy Car Showrooms. I didn't really like it here. The girls in the office were ok but the car salesmen were your stereotypical car salesmen – full of themselves! I had only been there a couple of weeks when a job appeared on the Town Hall bulletin (the only way to get a permanent job in the Council was to apply for any jobs that came up on the Council Internal Bulletin). It was for a Junior Clerk/Typist in the Planning Department. I was only learning to type at night school but my YTS Course Mentor said nothing ventured, nothing gained. I applied for the job and was invited to attend an interview. I was amazed when I was offered the job as I was the only applicant who wasn't proficient in typing. Later when I asked Brian, the Office Manager, why he had chosen me and not one of the other more experienced typists, he said I seemed mature for my age and he liked my attitude. I was quite confident in those days. Things were very different from Environmental |Health. I worked with a girl called Lynne and to say we were over-worked was an understatement. But because this was my first "proper" job I though that's the way things were. It is a myth to say Council jobs are easy. Yes, if you are the top of the pile but not if you are at the bottom – too many chiefs and not enough Indians. I did my best but there was so much to learn and it didn't help that Lynne was super efficient. I felt I came no where near to her! (I have later found out that this is a personality flaw of mine – always trying to be a perfectionist, instead of thinking she was 4 years older than me and much more experienced I felt I was lacking. Thankfully I am not like that now as I accept my good points and my bad points and don't try too hard to please everybody). With trying so hard at work I found college a real struggle. You got many assignments and after a hard days work the last thing I felt like doing was college assignments so I fell behind. I also remember getting a bad case of flue and I missed a couple of weeks at college. I started to feel panicky. I would be walking down the street and I would have to stop mid step as my heart would be pounding that fast and I felt so frightened. I didn't know what was happening to me. I would cry at the slightest thing. I felt trapped. I couldn't leave my job as I would be classed a failure and I wouldn't get another. I had to go to college or loose my job. Life wasn't supposed to be like this – after school everything was going to be perfect! My confidence was disappearing. I didn't want to go out with my friends. When I woke in the mornings I wished I could just turn over and go back to sleep and not have to deal with anything. Because this was my first experience with mental health I didn't know what was happening to me. I just felt I had no control over anything and I felt trapped and so very frightened.

Things went on like this for a few weeks but at least I was sleeping so I could go to work. Mum and Dad just thought I was run down from the flu and I didn't tell them how I was feeling. I just hoped for a miracle and everything would be ok.

Then one night I went to bed and sleep didn't come at all. The nightmare had begun. Only anyone who has suffered like this can truly understand. You <u>don't</u> sleep. I remember one "know it all" years ago saying "well you must sleep a bit you're just forgetting". No you lie there for hour after hour with all sorts of thoughts flooding through your mind. The more you try the harder it becomes. Even though I felt terrible the next day I went to work and didn't say anything to anyone about not sleeping. Getting through the day was horrendous. When I got home I had a nice relaxing bath but I dreaded going to bed. What if I couldn't sleep again – I couldn't go on like this! I was feeling like a zombie. So like a prisoner approaching the rack I climbed into bed. Sleep didn't come again. In the early hours of the morning I was past myself, I couldn't lie in that bed any more it was like torture. I went downstairs. Dad appeared in the kitchen. All of a sudden I broke down crying "I haven't been sleeping Dad its all too much, work, college – I can't cope". "This is what I have always dreaded" said Dad "that you or Stuart would be like me and suffer with your nerves". He sat down next to me and told me about his breakdown when he was 22 caused by stress at work. How he ended up in Winterton Mental Hospital (a much feared local mental hospital) the Institutional type of mental hospital now closed down. But after a couple of months he was well again and able to go back to work. He told me this but not to frighten me but to show me he knew how to handle mental illness. He asked me what was worrying me. I said work but mainly college as I had got so far behind and exams were looming. He asked if I stopped going to college would I be able to cope with work. I think so I said. He said he would try and sort it out with Brian, my Office Manager. I wasn't capable of sorting anything out. I went back to bed but I still didn't sleep. I realise now that mental illness isn't something that disappears overnight. I had taken weeks to get me into this state it would take weeks to get me well again.

Dad took some time off work and just sort of took over. I remember going to the Doctor with Dad but I don't think I was given any anti-depressants at that stage. But I do remember getting a sick note with the dreaded word "Depression" on it and I was told to take things easy. Dad had sorted things out with Brian my boss and when I returned to work I wouldn't have to attend college any more. I just felt like hiding away from the world but dad would make me go out. At first he would accompany me to the town, shops, supermarket etc. After a week or so he would make me go on my own. At the time I thought he was cruel for forcing me to do things I didn't want to do. But now I look back he was only doing it for my own good. You <u>have</u> to fight it. Take small steps and eventually it does get easier. You have to keep trying. The first time I left the house on my own I thought I was going to have a heart attack. I was sweating so much I could hardly make it past my own front door. But with hindsight I release if I hadn't made those first very, very hard but important steps my life would never have improved. Twenty years down the line I would be living in a cocoon with Mum and Dad. I would never have worked again, never got married, never experienced the sheer undiluted joy of having my two beautiful girls.

I remember at that time being terrified of seeing someone from work when I was out – what would they think! Certain things always stick in your mind and a receptionist at the Town Hall when she heard I was off with depression said, via another colleague, "What's a young girl like that have to be depressed about, if she can't cope with life at her age she never will!" That always sticks in my mind. This is just an example of the prejudice and ignorance people like me have to put up with every day.

To be honest as this was my first breakdown and the mildest by far I don't remember how I got well. I went for nights with no sleep. I was like a zombie but the doctor wouldn't give me sleeping tablets. By this stage I was on a mild anti-depressant but it wasn't really agreeing with me. My Nanna used to take sleeping tablets so she gave me some of hers. One night I took one. I still never slept but at about 5 in the morning I eventually dozed off. I had the most vivid nightmare that I thought I was awake and heads and hands were coming out of the bedroom wall to strangle me. I was screaming and shaking all over. Mum rushed into my bedroom and calmed me down saying I had had a nightmare. It was so vivid. That was my first and last experience with sleeping tablets.

I do have one clear memory of that time and that is of me stood at the top of the stairs at home wanting to throw myself down and try to end it (I realize now I wouldn't have died just probably broke something),. But something held me back.

My two close friends at the time, Claire and Angie, who are still two of my closest friends and have always stuck by me through the good and bad times, were really good with me, even though they were only 17 themselves and didn't really understand.

Prior to me getting ill me and Angie had booked a holiday to Lloret de Mar in Spain. So even though when I first became ill the thought of going filled me with horror, as I began to get slightly better it became something to focus on – getting well for my holiday.

After about 4 weeks I returned to work. Some people were a bit funny with me at first but time passes by and people forget. At this stage in my life I didn't realise I would always be vulnerable to mental health problems so I thought if I never worried and took on too much I would be ok.

I realise now that instead of dealing with problems or things that upset me I just put them to the back of my mind and concentrated on being happy. If nothing got to me I couldn't get ill again. My Dad hadn't so I couldn't.

By the time the holiday came round I was fine again and my outgoing personality was back again. (Even though I was a worrier at school, anyone who knew me well knew that I was quite chatty) and away from the constraints of school my personality had a chance to develop.

On holiday we had a great time. About half way through the holiday we met some boys that had been on our coach to Spain. We all got chatting and had a drink in a bar together. We met some girls and someone mentioned a party. It seemed like a good idea. We all went back to the boys apartment and had fun. After a while Angie wanted to go back to the hotel and I said I would be ok. There were still a few of us left but the boys were pouring the drinks and I quickly became drunk. Things became a bit hazy. I was sitting on the settee in the lounge and most of the others had left. I was thinking of leaving when one of the boys who had been flirting with me all night sat next to me. We began kissing and then he began tugging at my clothes. I said I was going but he took no notice and just became rougher. I tried to cry out but he put his hand over my mouth. My brain went into panic mode but outwardly I switched off. He raped me. I was only 17 and a virgin. This is the first time if have properly acknowledged that it did actually happen. I told no-one. So I know when my family and friends read this they will be shocked but I have to write it down and deal with it. When it was all over he left me and disappeared. I found the bathroom and locked the door. I cleaned myself up – there was blood between my thighs. Then I quickly found the front door and as I was leaving the boy who had raped me appeared and as I left he kissed me on the cheek and said bye. The crazy thing was I just accepted this, didn't accuse him, said bye and left. I thought no, I can't deal with rape I'll crack up again. I'll just forget it happened and get on with my life. I didn't dwell on it I just pushed it to the farthest recess of my mind.

However, when I returned to England it dawned on me that I could be pregnant. So without anybody knowing I made an appointment at the Family Planning Clinic. I didn't tell the nurse the story just that I had had unprotected sex. This was the 1980's and she never mentioned sexually transmitted diseases or AIDS. She asked me to do a pregnancy test and to be more careful next time. She asked if I wanted to go on the pill or if I wanted some condoms. I said no – I didn't even have a boyfriend! Thankfully the test was negative and in my mind the episode was closed never to be dredged up again. The reason I have included it in my book is it just goes to show what an effect the breakdown had had upon me. I was frightened of acknowledging anything traumatic in case it played on my mind and made me ill again.

I now realise 20 years later that you can't keep pushing things to the back of your mind. Eventually it will become clogged up with unsolved problems and it will explode (another breakdown).

Things went along fine for the next few months.

When I was 18 I started working a couple of nights a week in the Dolphin Centre bar. It was a council owned bar. I did it partly for extra money and because I thought it might be fun. I loved it! It was like part of my social life. The people were great and we had a laugh. One day somebody caught my eye. I won't name him, he knows who he is. We got talking in a nightclub after work one night and he said he was with someone but they were living separate lives due to split soon – they weren't married. That old chestnut and I swallowed it hook, line and sinker. We started a relationship albeit cloak and dagger. My confidence had been so rocked by past events that I accepted the crap way he treated me. My friends were always telling me to stop seeing him and that he was a selfish, self-centered bastard but I didn't want to over analyze the situation like I had in the past and make myself ill so I just plodded on letting him make a fool of me. Convincing myself that I loved him and him me

POLES APART

(love, ha! ha! I realise now that Billy is the only man that I have ever truly loved and who really loves me). Of course he didn't leave his girlfriend and we met in secret. Eventually she found out about us and they split up. But we were still not open about our relationship and we were still sneaking around. I vaguely recall him saying he didn't want to rub her nose in it and I accepted this like the fool I was. Things plodded on like this. I was 19 in the January and one day in May he asked to meet me. He said "You'd better sit down I've something to tell you – I got married yesterday!" I didn't even know he was still seeing her! He even suggested seeing each other occasionally but even I was not that stupid.

Not long after this I met Phil. He seemed so different. He wasn't particularly good looking but he treat me like a lady and seemed really kind and caring. I had gone purely for looks with my ex but as my Mum says "there's many a good looking nought" and this was so true.

I had been friendly with a Canadian girl called Tracy who worked at the Dolphin Centre bar. When she returned to Canada me and Angie made plans to go and see her. We flew from Manchester to Edmonton in Alberta via Toronto. Tracy met us at the airport and said she had a nice surprise for us. We had expected to stay with Tracy but one of her neighbors had gone on holiday for a week and they said we could stay in their house. Tracy and her parents lived in a very nice suburb of the city. The house, when we first saw it, reminded me of something out of Knots Landing. It was great having the house to ourselves. At the time the film "Dirty Dancing" had just come out and I bought the album and a bottle of "Paris" perfume at the airport. I just have to smell this scent and hear a track from the album and I am transported back to that magical holiday. The house was within walking distance of the West Edmonton Mall. Which, at that time, was the largest shopping mall in the world? I and Angie spent many a happy hour in there. There was a giant aquarium and you could go on a submarine ride. Tracy's friends were very hospitable. We got taken to an American football match and an ice hockey match. We saw the entire city. They threw parties in our honor. One particularly sticks in my mind. One of Tracy's friends lived alone in a bungalow/ranch style house. He had a hot-tub in his yard (garden). He had put a good spread of food on and plenty of booze! Alchopops were very fashionable at the time in Canada (they called them coolers) but were virtually unheard of in the UK. Because they taste like pop you don't recognise their strength. We were told there was a hot-tub and to bring our bathing costumes (July when we went is very hot in Alberta). We all ended up in the hot-tub and didn't need to get out very often as there were buckets of ice holding booze surrounding us.

When I eventually got out going to the toilet my legs were that wobbly from the drink I fell over – I didn't even release that I was that drunk! At the

POLES APART

end of the first week we went to Calgary for the weekend to attend the Calgary Stampede (Word famous rodeo). We had a fabulous time and Tracy returned to Edmonton on the Monday for work. I and Angie had bought unlimited travel tickets for the greyhound bus. Our plan was to go through the Rockies taking in Jasper and Banff National Parks and ending up in Vancouver. We did all of the above and the views of the Rockies were spectacular. When we stopped at Banff, a beautiful little town nestled in the Rockies we decided to make a day of it. We hired bikes to explore. We cycled for a while taking in the breathtaking scenery. We had gone far into the National park and were feeling a bit tired. We stopped to rest by a lake. We both stretched out on the grass next to our bikes and with the majestic mountains towering above us, nodded off. We were that naïve that we hadn't seen signs to be careful about snakes etc. There are also bears in the National Park. How dozy we were to have nodded off! When we came back from our travels on the greyhound we stayed a week at Tracy's and then it was time to go home. Me and Angie still keep in touch with Tracy and in 2005 she came up to Darlington to see us. Her husband is an executive with an oil company in Alaska and he had to come to England on business. He stayed down south and she traveled up north to see us. I met at the train station and within minutes it was as if we had never been apart. She's never changed – she's a wonderful person Tracy.

I was away for three weeks and when I came back I realised how much I had missed Phil. We had been dating quite steady for a few weeks when Phil booked a surprise trip for us to Bruges in Belgium. It was very romantic and I began to fall in love with Phil.

Phil was very fond of the good things in life and quite materialistic. But as I had a well paid job I also liked nice things so I didn't see any harm in this. I was only nineteen and Phil was twenty-five and he took me to some fabulous places and we had a great time. I was brought up not to take advantage of anyone so even though Phil earned more than me (he was at that time working off-shore as a Catering Manager on an oil rig) I still paid my way.

Phil had been a chef since he left catering college and he was sick of it. He wanted a career change and got the notion of becoming a pilot. He started having flying lessons and all of his money went on this. Phil was very intelligent and very strong-willed. When he set his mind on something nothing would get in the way. He passed his Private Pilots License Exams and set about getting his Commercial Pilots License.

He got on very well with the instructor at his flying school and one weekend he announced that they were chartering a sense twin-engine aircraft and flying to Rotterdam. I went with them and my heart was in my mouth a few times!

Prior to Phil starting his flying lessons he bought a cottage at Gainford, a village near Darlington. It was run-down and he was going to do it up and live in it eventually. I could easily have paid half the mortgage on my wages and I would have been keen but Phil had been financially wounded by a previous girlfriend so he wanted to buy the house solely. I kept my feelings to myself. I continued to be supportive to Phil while he continued with his quest to be a pilot. Phil didn't economise and still liked expensive meals out etc and although he was in debt I was increasingly running up my credit cards. I always believed that when he made it as a Pilot we would probably get married and be financially secure. I even bought a car on a bank loan and when Phil was home for two weeks at a time (he worked two on, two off on the rigs), he used the car quite a lot and I had to use the bus sometimes, although he never used buses.

.

For two years things had been going well at work since my last breakdown and I was now efficient and respected at my job. I had attended college again but this time it was for my typing, shorthand and secretarial qualifications. I passed all my exams with distinctions. There had been a restructuring and I and Lynne were now Word Processor Operators and our department was much larger. Typically of this department we were always very busy but I knew my job inside out by now and didn't mind as I am a hard and conscientious worker. Dad always said "Us Robbie's pride us on being good workers and not shirkers".

Prior to the restructure, Brian, the Office Manager, got a new job and left Darlington Borough Council. His position wasn't filled for a couple of months. Lynne and I did his job between us. Our departmental secretary Elaine became pregnant and wanted to do job-share. Lynne was offered the other half of Elaine's job and accepted. So Elaine became part-time secretary and Lynne was part-time secretary and part-time word processor operator. We didn't only do word processing we did many other duties. Then some time later Lynne applied for a new position in a different department and got the job. She left and I was offered to job share with Elaine and also be part-time word processor operator like Lynne had done – I accepted. Things were fine until Elaine went on maternity leave. I then had to do the secretarial post full-time (nb town hall secretaries have a lot of responsibility as you are secretary to a director and at the age of twenty I was very young to be doing this job!) So out of a team of three full-time members of staff there was only one left – me! We got a couple of temps in but I had to train them up. The job we did couldn't just be picked up overnight it had taken me three years to learn my job inside out. I was doing vast amounts of overtime. Things went on like this through the summer and although I was tired I was coping ok and things weren't getting on top of me.

Phil and I had booked a holiday to America for a month in the September. Phil was still doing really well with his flying. So we had reserved flights to Orlando airport in Florida. When we got there we were going to hire a twin-engine aircraft and fly around Florida and the Deep South of America so Phil could get some air miles in. Air time in the USA is much cheaper than in the UK. We had a fabulous but expensive holiday (Phil expected me to pay half his flying costs even though it was furthering his career and not mine. That holiday cost me personally in excess of four thousand pounds). We flew from Orlando to Miami, taking in the Florida Keyes on the way. Then we went to Tampa Bay on the Gulf Coast. Next it was Atlanta in Georgia, New Orleans, Nashville and last, but not least, Memphis. This was a dream for me as we went to Graceland – I love Elvis! So after working hard all summer I enjoyed my holiday and after one month away I went back to work totally relaxed.

Prior to me going to America our Director Robin had left the Authority. A new Director hadn't been appointed yet.

Also a girl called Annette who was roughly my age has been appointed full-time typist. I started to train her – she was very efficient. Elaine was back at work doing the part-time secretary post. A lady balled Gwen had been appointed part-time Word Processor Operator (the other half of my job).

When I returned to work we were really busy and as Annette had worked in other places besides Local Government she couldn't believe how much we were expected to do and how busy we were. I could cope with all this but everything changed when a new Director was appointed.

His name was Stephen and he came up a couple of weeks before he was due to start to meet everyone. His style of management was totally different. Whereas Robin was quite old fashioned and just let you get on with things the way they had always been done, Stephen seemed like a whirlwind to me with all the changes he wanted to implement. I felt panicky when I met him and out of my depth. (I would like to say that in time I would grow to like Stephen and I thought him a nice man but that was how I was feeling at the time).

After he had commenced work I remember mentioning work a lot to Phil and how it was getting to me but as nothing ever worried him he told me to "not let the bastards grind me down". Nobody ever took advantage of Phil but he was older and more experienced than me in the ways of the world. He had worked in different countries even. He told me to do my best and no more. He didn't see any alarm bells ringing because he didn't know me when I was 17.

POLES APART

I remember feeling really tired and listless. I was comfort eating and I didn't want to go out much. Everything was an effort. I particularly remember Christmas shopping in a department store called Binns in Darlington and dashing to the toilets to cry my heart out. The old feelings were returning "Please God not again" I remember thinking.

I remembered my Dad saying last time "You have to fight it Shell" so I went back to work and did my best and tried not to worry about the work piling up. I tried to focus on Christmas to cheer myself up. Shopping for gifts was an effort but I forced myself.

I remember saying to myself it won't happen again. I know my job inside out. I'm older, more experienced. I'm happy and I've got Phil now.

The day of our departmental Christmas lunch arrived. I got dressed up. (In those days I always kept slim, watched what I ate and wore nice clothes). For some reason I felt more positive that day. We had our lunch in a local restaurant. Then all the staff went back to the Town Hall. Elaine's daughter was poorly so she had taken the day off. I was secretary. The usual practice after a works Christmas lunch was for all the staff to congregate in one big office to have a drink together. So when everybody else was having a good time, Stephen wanted me to work – he wanted some letters typing urgently. I worked until home time and didn't have a drink. Just before I was due to go Elaine phoned, she said that her daughter had meningitis and she would be off work for the foreseeable future. I felt like I was sinking and I felt trapped like a caged animal with no way out. Of course I felt sorry for Elaine but all I could think was "Oh no I'll have to be secretary full-time and I can't cope".

I broke up from work the next day for the Christmas holidays. Christmas day dawned but I felt none of the joy of previous years. Just worry knawed away at my heart. We had lunch with my family and they were all so happy and loving I didn't want to go to Phil's family for tea. Of course I went because no-one knew how I was feeling – I was keeping all my thoughts and feelings to myself.   Hoping and praying that I wasn't becoming ill again.

Phil's brother Steve and his girlfriend Julia had bought the empty cottage next to Phil's at Gainford. They were both Catering Managers for Darlington Borough Council (I had met Phil through Steve). They had done their cottage up, no expense spared, and it looked beautiful. Phil, with my help had done up some of his cottage and we stayed there when he was home from the rigs. Steve and Julia were ok but not really my sort of people.   Steve and Julia were having food and drinks at their house. Phil's Mum, Julia's Mum and Julia's Mum's boyfriend had been there all day. The cottage looked like something out of a

POLES APART

"House and Garden" advert but there was none of the warmth of Mum's messy but welcoming home. I had always felt an outsider with Phil's family but as I loved Phil I turned a blind eye. They didn't seem to have my values which had been drummed into me and Stu by Mum and Dad from an early age. Mum and Dad always stressed to me not to judge a person by where they lived, how much money they had etc. but to judge the person for whom they were. Phil, Steven and Alan (Julia's Mum's boyfriend) went to the local pub for a couple of drinks. I felt so alone. They were all friendly in their own way but I wished I was at Mum's. I clearly remember one of Mum's friends turning up before we left. They were all laughing and having a good time. It was so safe and familiar there. When Phil came back from the pub we went next door to bed. I didn't let on to Phil how I was feeling. That night when Phil fell asleep I cried myself to sleep.

Roughly three days later Phil was due to go back to the oil rigs. I drove him to Middlesbrough were he got the bus to Aberdeen. I will never forget his face at the bus station. He kissed me, then cuddled me and said "Stop worrying about work it's not worth it". He had a last lingering look and then he was gone. That would be the last time he would see the old Michelle. I was becoming ill and our relationship was doomed. I started driving on the A66. It was about 11 pm and it was dark. All of a sudden I had to pull over onto the hard shoulder. My heart was beating so fast I thought I was having a heart attack. My palms were sweaty and I started to cry. "Please God not again". I knew then without a doubt that I had to do something and tell my parents.

When I got home Mum and Dad were watching TV. I asked them to switch it off as I had something to say. "My nerves are bothering me Dad but don't worry I'm going to sort things out at work – it's all been getting on top of me". "Good girl, look at how I keep on top of mine". Dad said. I was a failure. Why was I ill again? Why hadn't I learned the first time? Many years later and much water under the bridge I realise that once the stress has built up to this level there is little you can do to stop yourself becoming ill – it is an illness.

It was to be another five years before I would be diagnosed with bi-polar disorder (Manic Depression). That's why when I look back I don't feel a failure. I had, and have, an illness. Most of the time I am fine like most people but put under excessive amounts of stress and I will become ill without a doubt. I used to feel it was my entire fault and that I was a weak person. But now I feel the opposite. I think I am a strong person to have this illness and overcome the great hurdles that life has thrown at me.

Going back to that night. I went to bed as it was late. I slept and felt a little better as I had decided

POLES APART

to ask for my old job back (full-time Word Processor Operator). As I was only part-time secretary and part-time Word Processor Operator and there was more than enough work I thought it was an easy solution to get a part-time secretary to cover the other half of Elaine's job. I thought with what had happened to me at seventeen due to stress at work they would agree rather than let me get ill again.

Next day I went to see my Administrative Manager, Ray, and told him the job was too much and was getting on top of me. I asked if I could have my old job back. He replied that it would be a bit difficult, as there was no funding. Elaine would be back soon and things would be fine. Other things were said but that was the jest of it.

Deflated I got through the rest of the day but I was sinking fast. I couldn't concentrate. I typed a letter and checked it eight times for errors – I was becoming paranoid. There was so much work to do. As I had been there the longest and had the most experience staff would come to me if there were problems. I remember one of the officers shouting that a letter had been in the typing tray for days and instead of fighting back and saying we were understaffed I got tears in my eyes. I remember Gwen and Annette also being stressed out with the work but they didn't have a mental illness.

That was a Friday and on the night I was due to have some friends round as I was having a naughty knickers party. I left work early and got home before anyone else. I just sat and cried for about an hour. I covered my red eyes with make-up and said I was getting a cold to my friends. I drank quite a bit that night to try and blot everything out. But although when I went to bed I slept, I woke up in the middle of the night in a mad panic. My heart was beating out of control and I was sweating like mad. I did not go back to sleep I just lay in the darkness terrified.

It was my birthday the next day. I was 22. Me, Mum, Dad, Stu and his new girlfriend, Sandra, (who was my age) all went out for a meal in a nice restaurant. The food stuck in my throat I was so chewed up. After the meal Stuart and Sandra were going to a nightclub and asked me to go. I could not go the way I was feeling but I remember looking at them and feeling so jealous and resentful. I thought they are only my age and they have never suffered like this. I should be happy and carefree like them, why am I cursed?

I returned home with Mum and Dad and we had a talk. I don't think at that stage they were overly worried because my Dad had only had one breakdown and never got that ill again. That's one of their problems always thinking I am like my Dad. I am in certain ways but I am still me. My Dad was like many people who have one breakdown, get well and never have another breakdown.   I am different; I have a serious mental illness. I will always have this and I have to watch how much stress I am putting on myself.

It is only at this stage of my life that I count myself lucky with my illness as it could be a lot worse. A lot of people don't understand Manic Depression. They think it means that you are always depressed. This is nothing of the sort. It means that there is a chemical imbalance in your brain and one day you could be on top of the world, the next day deeply depressed. Some suffers go weeks on high then weeks on a low. Every sufferer has different symptoms. Most need constant medication to rectify the imbalance so they are neither too high or too low just stable and on an even keel. All three of my breakdowns have been caused by severe stress in the workplace. Now I have not worked for ten years I have not had another breakdown. Some winters I am not as happy as I am in the summer but I wouldn't say I am depressed. I suffer more with the "high" side of my illness. While feeling high is a good feeling, being too high can be dangerous. When I had my oldest daughter Kristy I went high (I had been deeply, deeply depressed for about two years beforehand), I loved my child and couldn't get enough of life. I still hadn't been diagnosed with suffering from Manic Depression and didn't realise that I was ill. Luckily I came down of my own accord or I could have ended up very ill and even psychotic.

Also I have come to realise that excess alcohol doesn't agree with me. I went to Bennidorm for a week's holiday with my friends last year. I had a great time and got on a high. All the very late nights, excess alcohol and not eating properly took its toll. When I came home I was very high and just kept getting higher. Luckily I went to the doctor before I became too ill and she prescribed some strong medication to bring me down. I still had to stay at Mum and Dads for a week to get my head sorted. I was too ill to cope with my darling girls. Billy had to take over. After one week I was ok again.

Back to the night of my birthday. I went to bed that night but at least I slept. I knew that I was deeply depressed at that stage but as long as I could sleep I could go to work and function properly.

The next day was Sunday. On that Sunday I went to bed and sleep never came. I was hurtling into the deep black tunnel again.

I went to work the next day. Annette commented that I looked worn out and I started crying. She told me to go home and take things easy, have a couple of days off she said. Bless her she was only trying her best – if only it were that easy. I remember sitting on the bus and feeling doomed.

By this stage in my life my brother Stu also worked on the oil rigs and he was home with my Mum when I got in "I got sent home Mum" I said. I could tell she was worried sick.

The pattern was repeated like last time. I wasn't sleeping, I couldn't eat. This time Dr. Young put me on anti-depressants but anyone who has ever taken them will tell you they take weeks to kick in. Also extreme amounts of stress at work had made me ill. How was a little pill going to cure me when the stress was still there?

A week had gone by and I still hadn't slept. My Mum said she was going to take me out to a quiet pub to meet some friends of hers. She said if I had a good drink it might help me to sleep. I got drunk. She had to help me to bed. Whilst I was drinking I felt slightly better. I went to sleep as soon as my head hit the pillow. I was in a drunken sleep having a vivid dream about work when I woke up in a mad panic with my heart beating like mad. I looked at the bedside clock, I had only been asleep two hours. I lay in the darkness feeling so frightened and low. Phil wouldn't want me like this. I was a wreck. All my confidence had vanished. My hair was dull. My complexion was spotty and pasty. I didn't even put my face on – something I always did normally. I usually took a pride in my appearance. I was so down nothing seemed to matter.

The next day was Friday. I felt unbelievably low that day. I now realise many years later that as I was deeply depressed the excess drink had sent me plummeting down even further.

On the Saturday Mum and Dad were off work. They said I couldn't stay in the house on my own. They were going out to meet their friends for a drink and said it would do me good to go with them. It was like I had lost my identity. I was like a child. I know they were only going it for my own good but I was a 22 year old career woman being told where to go, what to do and what to eat (Mum was making me her lovely filling meals, which I had avoided since starting work as although they tasted fabulous they weren't kind to the waistline). I had struggled with my weight for years and now I was going to end up fat. I was bitter with the unfairness of life.

Whilst on the subject of the unfairness of life, when I was deeply depressed I was so jealous of my brother Stuart. I love him dearly but whilst I was ill I couldn't help but compare my life to his. In my eyes he had everything and he was truly blessed. He is drop-dead gorgeous looking. He has lovely dark hair, dark brown eyes and olive skin (I burn easily). Our grandmother (paternal) was half Italian and it has come out in Stu. He was academically average at school and nobody put any pressure on him to do well. He just breezed through school, always really popular and he never worried about anything. Although he never really tried at school to get any qualifications at that point when I was ill he was working on the rigs and earning good money. He had never had his heart broken – he was usually the heart breaker! He was tall and had a fabulous muscular physique. He had never struggled with his weight. He ate like a pig and never put an ounce on. I used to think how can one child be so blessed and the other cursed. Of course all these negative thoughts were whilst I was ill (it is a factor in deep depression to think everyone is more talented, better etc than you). I now realise that everyone has their own special qualities and I have mine just like Stu. I love Stu deeply. He is a great brother and we have always been really close. I know I can always depend on him.

Referring back to Saturday. We went to a pub then back to Mum and Dad's friends, Paul and Margaret's house. I had always got on with them and thought them lovely. But I could see it in their faces and their actions that they didn't understand. I knew exactly what they were thinking "Michelle had everything going for her why does she do this to herself?" An example of how people think like this is the following exhibit from the News of the World, Feb 5, 2006 "How sad that beautiful actress Lindsay Lohen is in hospital after cutting herself. She has everything going for her. Why can't she see it?" Ria Jones, Denbigh – the answer to this question is mental illness and stress. Some of the most talented people in the world suffer from mental illness. A lot of people think it is just weak-minded people with no self-discipline. How wrong they are.

When we returned home it was quite late. As I had had quite a lot to drink I went straight to bed. I didn't sleep. I heard Mum and Dad saying that Phil would be home soon as although it would be a shock for him to see me like this, with his help I would get better.

All of a sudden I became so angry. I started punching myself. When Mum and Dad had retired to bed I went downstairs and found Dad's whiskey bottle. I drank two glasses straight down, even though I hate the taste of whiskey. I went back to bed. "Why should Phil see me like this, I'd rather be dead, I'd rather he remember the old Michelle" (now I know I suffer from Bi-polar disorder I realise that the excess drink had made me psychotic and out of touch with reality). I never thought about the people I loved like Mum, Dad and Stu I just wanted the immense pain to go away. Without thinking I went into the bathroom and found some tablets in the bathroom cabinet and I washed them down with stardrops. I crawled into bed and waited to die. I must have dozed off with all the drink and pills.

All of a sudden it was morning. Sunlight was coming through the curtains. I woke up. At first I didn't remember that I'd done the previous night. Then it all came flooding back. I couldn't believe I was still alive. I told no-one what I'd done. I still thought I would die but maybe that night. I was in a state of madness.

POLES APART

Phil rang the next day. Dad answered, gave Phil a short greeting and then handed me the phone. On the rigs you can't ring all the time. This was the first time I'd heard his voice since he'd been away. I can't remember exactly what he said but it was along the lines of "I was worried something like this would happen, you take a couple of weeks off and you'll be as right as rain – I love you". I hardly uttered a word. Oh no what had I done! Phil's words had shocked me into reality. I was dying – I didn't want to die. I wanted to see Phil, I loved him. What about Mum, Dad and Stu – I loved them too. I started to get hysterical "Mum, Dad phone an ambulance I've got to go to hospital". "Why" they said. "I'm dying" I said. "Don't be silly, of course you're not dying" they said. I didn't mention pills or star drops, I was ashamed. They thought it was my illness talking.

I was sobbing hysterically on the bed but Mum just thought I needed to get it out of my system. When you are mentally ill one of the symptoms is thinking all sorts of things are wrong with you – you can become a bit of a hypochondriac.

That night my Mum took me to see my Aunty Linda, my lovely Godmother. My Dad went for a drink with my Uncle Alf. When we walked home in the dark that night I clearly remember seeing a man walking a little puppy near the park. I remember thinking if only I hadn't taken the tablets and star drops I would get a puppy of my own. I would be able to get out and get well. I looked at Mum and Dad – I loved them so much, but I knew it was too late, the damage was done – I was dying. For days after taking the star drops all I could taste was this and in my madness I thought it was poisoning my system and I would have a slow death. It was only when I was well months later that I realised it was only working its way out of my system and it wouldn't kill me and whatever the tablets had been they couldn't have been harmful as if they were going to kill me I would have been dead by then. But one of the factors in any mental health problem is loosing touch with reality and this is what had happened to me. So years later whilst writing this book, or even six months down the line when I was well again, I can see things clearly. At the time my mind was so mixed up with irrational thoughts nobody but me could understand.

Phil came home on the Friday. I was upstairs when he arrived. Mum or Dad – I can't remember which, called me down. But what I clearly remember is the look of disappointment on his face as if I'd let him down. He suggested a drive out and even though I was terrified of leaving the house I agreed. Once in the car we were like strangers. The atmosphere was terrible. We drove along in silence and then I'll remember these words till my dying day "This has never happened to anyone in my family but I'll stick by you this time but don't let it happen again" he said. I never said a word – I couldn't. It was as if a hand had plunged into my chest and ripped my heart out.

The man I thought I loved more than anything. Who in my madness I had even tried to kill myself for so he didn't se me like this was just a self-absorbed shallow nothing and the people who truly loved me for me (Mum, Dad and Stu) would be left to pick up the pieces when I died. Phil would just walk away. Phil thought it was a weakness and my own entire fault. He and his family are like countless others who don't even try to understand mental health and that's why there has always been stigma attached and always will be until peoples attitudes change.

He took me to his Mum's house and she was very wary of me. She said something along the lines of "Oh well you'll be back at work in a couple of weeks" as if I had a bad cold. I couldn't wait to go home I felt so uncomfortable.

As he was driving me home he said something along the lines of "Oh Shell why did this have to happen I love you and <u>wanted</u> to marry you". It was as if the old Michelle had died and the new one wasn't good enough to marry.

That evening Phil wanted to go through to Gainford to have a drink in the local pub with Steve and Julia. Of course the thought of this filled me with horror but Mum and Dad said it would do me good. "You'll never get better stuck in this house, you have to fight it" Dad said. Whilst I was getting ready upstairs I heard Dad having a chat with Phil about his breakdown at 22 and how he'd been fine since. He was more or less implying that we'll get Shell through this and she'll be fine forever after.

Phil's attitude got a bit better after that and he seemed more caring. We drove to the pub at Gainford and I was in a state. Prior to becoming ill I was still working a couple of nights a week in the Dolphin Centre and Steve was my boss. This was the first time they'd seen me since Christmas. I could tell they were shocked by my appearance. Prior to becoming ill I was always immaculately dressed; I washed my hair every day and always wore make-up. I dieted constantly to keep slim so Phil would be proud of me. Image meant a lot to Phil. I had lost weight as I couldn't eat and I looked gaunt. I think I might have put a little make-up on but I didn't look anything like I usually did. Steve and Julia didn't know what to say. Phil just started talking about something to break the silence. A couple of their friends joined us and Julia sat next to me "You are really lucky to have Phil. Steve has told me if it was him he would have dumped you but Phil has said he'll stick by you – you should count your blessings!"

I know they were talking about me behind my back and saying "Poor Phil to have a 'nutter' for a girlfriend". I didn't tell Mum or Dad anything anybody said I just kept it to myself.

POLES APART

As the cottage was only half finished, we did some painting while he was off. Then Phil went back to the rigs. I could tell it was a relief to get away from me.

Annette from work had shown herself to be a good friend. She would ring and ask how I was and not to worry about work. My boss and section manager never picked up the phone or wrote a letter. I know the way the Town Hall thinks. I was a nuisance – it was inconvenient to have to cover my job. They couldn't have cared a less about me – I was only a number. Never in a million years would they have attached any blame on themselves. They had put that much stress on a 22 year old as to give them a nervous breakdown. The willing horse gets all the work but is easily forgotten.

Annette had told me they had two temps in to do the work. I know I was doing the workload of at least two people. Julia, a temp, who would later become a permanent member of staff, was twelve years older than me and had worked in many other places, couldn't believe how much I was expected to do before I was ill. I didn't find this out until I returned to work many months later.

One day Annette rang me and said the girls were going for a pizza at lunchtime for someone's birthday. "Did I want to go?" she asked. Mum persuaded me. I got a taxi and I remember wishing it would crash so I didn't have to go. When I got there it was so strange. Nobody knew what to say to me. Only Annette was normal. As the lunch wore on a couple of the others, Elaine and Ann, became a bit chatty and as we were leaving Pizza Hut, which was near the Town Hall, they linked my arm "Come on down to work everybody would love to see you!" I was petrified. They steered me towards the Town Hall. Nobody was friendly. The reception staff looked at me with strange expressions on their faces. Once we got to the third floor where I worked I saw a couple of colleagues. They had half smiles on their faces and didn't show any concern. If I had been off with a serious physical illness they would have all been round me like bees around a honey pot but as I was 'depressed' I didn't warrant any sympathy only contempt.

When we entered my office, which was a bit like an open plan office with the Director's office attached, Stephen, my boss, was there. The look on his face said it all! He was like Phil; he thought mental illness was a weakness. He didn't ask how I was, just when I was coming back to work. I looked around the office and I felt so panicky I could almost taste my own fear. I got out of there as quickly as I could and got a taxi straight home – I couldn't get home quick enough. I knew that I would never set foot in the Town Hall again. Mum had popped out for something and I lay on the bed and broke my heart. I was frightened of dying and going to hell as I'd tried to commit suicide. I was terrified of leaving Mum, Dad and Stu (Phil didn't fit into the equation – I had stopped loving him after his cruel words and actions) and a couple of good friends. My Dad once said you are truly lucky if you get a couple of good friends in a lifetime and there were never more true words spoken. I wanted to get better and be like everyone else getting on with their lives but I couldn't. I was dying – only no-one knew it. I wasn't even taking my medication as what was the point I couldn't get better the damage was done.

Every day was like torture. It was like someone was sticking a knife in my heart. Although I was still deeply depressed I wasn't psychotic. I was sleeping by this stage and I could see everything I would miss by dying. All the love and understanding by Mum, Dad and Stu (even though sometimes Dad's love is tough love – he did it with best intentions). If you just lie down and give up with this illness it will beat you – you have to pick yourself up even though it is so hard and just keep trying. That's why it is so hard because it's down to the individual. With a serious illness such as cancer it is up to early diagnosis and the skill of the doctors and surgeons who treat you. In many ways it is out of your control.

Dad booked a weekend trip to London for himself, Mum and me. I dreaded going. But away from home I felt slightly better. I liked the vastness of London and no-one knowing who you were. On the negative side it was breaking my heart to see how Mum and Dad were trying and looking to the future, when I knew I wouldn't be there.

One day my Aunty Linda and Uncle Alf (now departed – God bless him he was a lovely man) visited. My Aunty Linda understood as she had suffered with her nerves herself. But Uncle Alf was so laid back nothing ever stressed him. I know he was only being nice and trying to help me – he didn't have a nasty bone in his body – but he said something along the lines of "Go to the beach Shell and look at all the sand. We are all just like grains of sand, here one day and gone the next. Nothing is worth worrying about". A short while later I said I was going to the shop in my car. But when I reached the shop I just kept driving. I drove into the countryside. Eventually I stopped and looked around. I wished I could start again and have no worries. I know I was only being paranoid but I used to think all my family and friends talked about me and didn't understand me. Why did this have to happen to me I asked myself. I am not a bad person; all I've ever tried to do is my best and be a good person. Although we didn't have a lot of material things growing up Mum and Dad always taught us the right values – sadly values that I think are lacking in a lot of society nowadays. Respect your elders, never lie or cheat, good manners, don't think anybody is better or below you, treat each individual on their merits (one of Dad's sayings was "Don't forget those you meet on the way up as they are the ones you'll see on the way down").

POLES APART

I started to feel deep resentment and hated myself. It's not fair why I couldn't have been more like Stuart. I sat in the car for ages with all sorts of jumbled thoughts going through my head. I started to cry about the unfairness of life. I knew Mum and Dad would be worried but I just had to get out of the house. I couldn't face going home and having another lecture. I found a call box and rang Angie. I started sobbing "Angie can I come and see you?"

Ian was working away (they had recently got engaged). She suggested I stay the night. She would ring Mum and Dad. It would give us a break from each other.

Angie was really good with me even though half I was talking was an incoherent jumble. At some point that evening she was sick and when I asked her if she was ok her face took on a sad look "I didn't want to tell you Shell but you might find out off someone else – I'm pregnant!" I know she was overjoyed but she was such a god friend that she didn't want to rub my nose in it. She must have thought everything in my life is going great and look at poor Michelle. I would have felt the same if the roles were reversed.

Now I am well I believe you should count your blessings and never get envious of other people. You never know when the hand of fate will intervene and your life will be turned upside down.

Everyone has their crosses to bear – some more than others! I am saying this because three years down the line from this day, I have met Billy and Angie is pregnant again. Travis, her dear little boy, will be about three. She is expecting twins this time and sadly looses one early in pregnancy. When she is about six months pregnant she goes into labor prematurely and has lovely Matthew. His life hangs in the balance but he doesn't die. He is severely brain damaged and has cerebral palsy. Angie and Ian are very special people. He sadly died when he was only seven. He must be in heaven with his twin brother Liam. Angie and Ian aren't bitter and just get on with life for the sake of the lovely Travis and the cute Connor (Angie had Connor when Matthew was about 2).

Angie is completely different in nature to me. She is very calm and sensible whilst I am a bit scatty. When I first met her when we were both 11 and had just started long field I didn't like her! She has two older brothers who were really popular and good looking and she was so confident and knew all the older kids – I was so envious. I had been separated from my friends who had gone into different classes and was feeling like a duck out of water. Within a few weeks of being at Long field I did start to like her but Angie wasn't as swotty as me so we didn't become close until we had left school. In the summer holidays straight after leaving school I had a job delivering leaflets and I bumped into Angie. She gave me a hand to do them and we really got on. As I have previously said, my personality didn't really come out until I had left school. We started to socialize along with Claire and a couple of other friends. Angie has never been one for going out a lot so we didn't live in each others pockets.

She is very caring, loyal and has a heart of gold. I am scatty, Claire is even scattier and Angie is level headed. I know it sounds a weird combination for friendship but we all love and respect one another, have been friends for over twenty years and never bitch or fall out.

She didn't go to college she went on an YTS like me. She eventually got a job at Press Construction but the pay was so poor I suggested her coming to work at the Dolphin Centre with me. She loved it and through the Dolphin she met her lovely husband Ian.

One day Annette came to the house and discussed going back to work for a couple of days a week. Mum and Dad thought it a good idea. I agreed even though I was petrified. I went for a drive with Phil on the Sunday, the day before I was due back at work. When he dropped me back at home in the evening he seemed very pleased that with my going back to work the old Michelle would soon return.

I watched TV with Mum and Stu – Dad was out. I was desperately sad that this was my last night alive. I was never going back to the Town Hall. I was dying anyway so tomorrow I was going to finish the job properly. I went to my room with a leaden heart. How I wished things were different. I got into bed and cried as it my heart was breaking – which it was! I got under the covers so no-one could hear. I didn't think I would sleep but exhaustion got the better of me.

I awoke when I heard my Dad's alarm going off for work. All of a sudden I was transported back to a different time, when as a teenager I would wake up to the same sound, lie in the snug warmth for a few minutes before Dad would knock on my door and say "Shell time to get up". Dad and I were always the first to rise in those days (Mum and Stu liked their lie-ins) and if I had a French test that day he would test me on my verbs. Although I didn't really like school, when I woke I always wondered what the day would bring and I had a bright future ahead if I tried hard and did well.

I wanted to stay in the nice warm bed but death wasn't going to come to my comfy bed. It was going to happen elsewhere and it was going to be ugly, cold and brutal.

I got dressed and had a last look around my room. I could tell by Dad's face that he was hoping for more a change in my appearance. I wasn't what you could call overly smart and I hardly had any make-up on. He told me that he was proud of me for going back to work and he couldn't wait to see me after work that night. I looked at his face and drank in his features – this would be the last time I would see my Dad I told myself.

I got a bus to the town centre. Then instead of going to the Town Hall like everybody thought, I got on another bus to take me to the train station. When I arrived at the station there were lots of coaches and station personnel saying there was a dispute and no trains were running. The coaches were taking people to their destinations. I didn't even have a plan in mind but I had to get out of Darlington quickly as Mum, Dad or Phil would ring the Town Hall that morning and if I wasn't there they would know I had gone missing. I got on the first bus and it was going to Newcastle. As the bus left the town I looked around. This would be the last time I would see Darlington.

There were two girls sitting in front of me giggling about something. They were dressed like they were going to work. Oh god I thought I wished I was them with my whole life ahead of me. I remember thinking nobody knows what's going on in someone's mind. Here I am sitting on this bus looking like I am going to work or shopping when I am going to take my own life. Nobody could ever guess by looking at me.

When I arrived at Newcastle I wandered around aimlessly for a while, then I decided to get on the Metro. I didn't know where I was going to get off. The end of the line was Whitley Bay.

When I arrived at Whitley Bay, a small seaside town, I headed for the seafront. It was a sunny day and quite warm. There were quite a few people about with their dogs and some with children – how I wished I could swap places with them.

I was walking along the edge of the cliffs. I started crying and looking up to the sky to heaven. I was convinced I was going to hell as I was taking my own life. I remember shouting "Nanna, help me, I wish I could be with you in heaven (even though Nanna had committed suicide I thought she had led such a self-less life God would have forgiven her).

I wandered about for a bit more but became panicky. I didn't have a watch on but knew it must be afternoon and they would be looking for me. I had to do it soon and do it right. They would all know why I had come here and I couldn't stand to see the looks on their faces.

I didn't jump off the cliff. I lay down and sort of rolled down. I ended up at the bottom in deep mud. I didn't hurt myself. Oh no I thought I can't do anything right. I was face down in the mud and wondered why my life had come to this. Somebody called an ambulance.

Of course the paramedics had seen it all before. Once they had established that I was a stranger to the town, on my own and walking at the edge of the cliffs, they knew that I had tried to top myself. Then their attitudes changed. I was a nuisance, a time waster. I was seriously ill but in their eyes I was just a nutter heading for the loony bin.

They took me to the local hospital. A couple of the nurses were funny and a couple was ok. I was checked over and put in a side ward. They were waiting for a phyciatrist to see me. One eventually came. Even though I had been ill for weeks this was the first time I had seen one. He spoke to me for a few minutes and then he went. I don't remember what he said.

In the meantime Mum, Dad and Phil arrived. Dad looked so sad; Mum was crying and happy that I was alive. Phil didn't say anything. They wanted to commit me but Dad, with the support of my Doctor, agreed that I would be better at home and Mum was going to take time off work to look after me.

The weeks dragged on with not much change in me. Phil was studying for his pilots exams and I didn't see much of him. Even though he was off for two weeks at a time he never offered to look after me. Mum was the one who had to do it and not even get paid from work. Phil thought about one person – himself!

One Saturday he suggested going out for a drive. I agreed. We ended up at Barnard Castle, a small market town near Darlington. We went into a café. The atmosphere was very tense. On the way home Phil hardly said two words. When we arrived home to my house we started to argue over my attitude. He said something along the lines of it had been months and he saw no improvement and was it always going to be like this. More words were said. I said I was going and didn't want to see him again. That was what he had wanted all along for me to finish with him. Then he could have a clear conscience. He could tell people he had tried but I had finished it. He drove away in my car.

There was nobody in the house. I sat in my room and broke my heart. Some days I used to think I couldn't possibly have any tears left. I wasn't crying because we had split up. I had stopped loving Phil a long time ago. I cried for the mess that was my life. I still thought I was dying.

Mum and Dad cam home soon after that and we all hugged and cried. Phil brought the car round, dumped it and drove off with his Mum or brother. Dad was looking out of the window but he couldn't see which.

Mum and Dad were aware that I had been paying for the car but they were shocked that I had paid the insurance and the car tax also. They also saw him in a different light now. Eventually when I became well one of my friends told me to take Phil to court for a percentage of the house profits (house prices had raised dramatically). I was on

POLES APART

the Poll Tax Register for Gainford and although I didn't pay the mortgage I paid for other things. I was in debt through living the high life with Phil. Also I had helped him to do the cottage up. But I had said I didn't want anything off Phil. I had totally been there for him when he needed me but he hadn't been for me. Money was his god - let him go and worship it.

A couple of weeks later the post arrived. Mum was out of the house and I was on my own. There was a letter addressed to me from the Town Hall. I opened it. They wanted me to see the Occupational Health doctor at the Town Hall. "Oh no I can't set foot inside there again". I ran upstairs to my room and hastily wrote a letter. I said all the things I was feeling. That I loved Mum, Dad and Stu so much but I had taken the tablets and stardrops and I was dying. There was no hope for me but I would always love them. I left it where they would find it, got my handbag and car keys. Then I left the house.

I started driving. I didn't know where I was going. I just kept driving. I felt safe inside my car. Eventually I ended up at Whitby. I wandered around for a bit. I desperately wanted to hear Mum's voice so I rang home from a phone box. "Oh love where you have been, we are so worried. Ray and Elaine are here from work to see you!" I hung up without saying another word.

I wandered around for a bit more. It was becoming dark. I booked into a bed and breakfast. The landlady showed me to my room. When she left I shut the curtains and got into bed. I kept my clothes on – I didn't have any nightware. I didn't sleep much. My heart was so heavy.

Next morning I checked out. The landlady had asked me some questions. I told her my car had broken down that's why I had to stay overnight and had no change of clothes. I told her I would collect my car that day and return home.

I got in my car and just started driving. I ended up at Scarborough. The previous day was more or less repeated. I wandered aimlessly around Scarborough until it was late afternoon and then I looked into another bed and breakfast. I stayed in bed in my room all night. I didn't eat or watch TV. I just lay in the poetal position and cried.

On the third day I ended up at Bridlington. I was missing Mum and Dad so much it was like a physical pain. I was wandering down a street and I saw a phone box. I had to hear one of their voices. I rang the number. It was picked up almost immediately by Mum. The heartbreak and sadness in her voice was so evident. I didn't speak I just hung up. I booked into the nearest bed and breakfast I could find even though it was only lunchtime. I got to my room and got into bed and under the covers. I cried until I was in a state of complete exhaustion and I just lay in the bed feeling numb.

On the fourth day I drove out of Bridlington and I was on a road leading to York. I came to a village and stopped to buy a drink. I knew I would be classed as missing so on impulse I bought a local newspaper "the Northern Echo". I waited until I was on the outskirts of the village before I pulled over again and opened the paper. There it was in print that I was missing. It gave details of who I was and that I was "depressed".

I carried on driving. Once I was on the main road leading to York again I was flashed to stop by a police car. I knew they would have my registration number as I was classed as a missing person. They asked me a few questions and then let me go on my way. I was amazed they hadn't taken me home.

All of a sudden it hit me like a thunderbolt that I wanted them to take me home. Even if I was dying I wanted to tell them everything and spend whatever time I had left with the people I loved – my family.

I reached the outskirts of York and found a phone box. I rang my brother Stu. I knew he wouldn't be annoyed with me. I knew Mum and dad loved me but I didn't know how upset they would be with me for letting everyone down and worrying them.

When he answered I could hardly talk for crying "Just come home Shell, we all love you and we'll do anything to help you".

I drove back home still ill and deeply depressed but determined to tell them everything so that least I could die at home with them around me.

It was getting dark when I arrived at Stu's (by this time he was living with his girlfriend, Sandra, in a house they had bought). He enveloped me in his arms while I sobbed my heart out. I was emotionally drained. "I'm putting you to bed, we'll talk tomorrow. I'll let Mum and dad knows you've arrived safely and I'll take you to see them tomorrow" Stu said.

He had made up a camp bed for me in his living room. I changed into one of Sandra's nighties and got into the snug bed by the fire. He made me a bite to eat and a hot drink. Then Stu and Sandra went to bed. They had just got some kittens and before he went out of the room he placed them on the bed. I thought they would just jump off and start playing as kittens do but no they snuggled into me and stayed there all night.

I will never forget that night. I suddenly felt safe after months of feeling frightened and alone. With the help of my family I was going to see a doctor, tell him/her everything and have a thorough physical to see what damage I had done. I was so very, very ill when I took the tablets and star drops

POLES APART

I didn't blame myself anymore. If, and when, I died I would be surrounded by my family and hopefully God would forgive me and I wouldn't go to hell. Once I had come to this decision, I slept like a baby, co-coned in the warmth of the fire and the purring of the kittens sending me to a peaceful sleep after nights of torture.

I was so apprehensive about seeing Mum and Dad but we all collapsed into each others arms and sobbed our hearts out.

I started at the beginning and told them about the tablets and stardrops. How for months I had thought I was dying and that's why there wasn't a vast improvement in me. That everyday from waking to going to bed that was all that was on my mind.

They listened and didn't condemn me but Dad said "love if it was going to kill you it would have by now". I would like to say that I believed him and I suddenly felt better again. It was to be a few more months before I was totally well again.

Dad agreed to accompany me to my Doctors the next day and get her to give me a physical to put my mind at rest. As I was still ill I knew they would see I was dying but at least it was out in the open and all my family knew how I was feeling.

My Aunty Ann (not real Aunty but I had known her since I was a baby and I was very fond of her) came over to see me. She told Mum and Dad that she had heard of a wonderful private hospital that specialized in Adult Mental Health. Sadly, the fees were astronomical and we couldn't afford it.

That is another factor in any health problem – mental or physical. Whilst I know money isn't everything and after everything I have gone through I am not materialistic. When you are ill money can get you the best possible care.

Of course Dr. Young agreed to look me over and she agreed with Mum and Dad that there was nothing physically wrong with me. She said she would get me an emergency appointment with a phyciatrist. Once home again I still wasn't convinced but instead of hiding my thoughts I said them out aloud "But she couldn't see my internal organs I may have damaged them" I said. For my peace of mind Dad suggested me paying to see a private doctor and have a thorough physical. I did go on to have this. It cost about 70 pounds and lasted one hour. He still didn't put my mind at rest.

It was more like a gradual process of getting well. I would say the crucial factor was work. My Administrative Manager, Ray and Elaine came out to visit me. They asked if I would consider going back to work part-time. No stress would be put on me.

POLES APART

I decided to give it a go and go back to work, mornings only. Prior to my going back to work my Aunty Ann had found about a lady who did "cognitive therapy". She lived in a small market town near Darlington called Richmond. She had a good reputation. We enquired about the service, costs etc. She wasn't that expensive and I decided to go for a trial visit. My other Nanna (Dad's Mum), who I would like to say I loved dearly, gave me some money towards my therapy. By this stage I had seen a phyciatrist a few times, and whilst I am definitely not racist, (I have a lovely friend called Bena who is Indian, and her beautiful little daughter Chloe is Kristy's best friend) both phyciatrists were foreign, probably of Asian descent. I could hardly understand what they were saying. How can you open your heart and soul if you can't make yourself understood!

As I have said previously, I still thought I was dying but I was willing to make a go of whatever time I had left.

On the Saturday before I was due to go back to work Mam and I went shopping. I got some new clothes for work. By this stage I had put on a lot of weight but I wasn't bothered – I would have put on five stone to have my old life back. I had my hair done and got some new make-up. We had a nice day and how I was coping was to imagine that if I knew I wasn't dying how would I act. I was pushing my dying negative thoughts to the back of my mind. This was possible during the day when I was busy but more difficult at night. I was sleeping ok but would have disturbed dreams and some panic attacks. Even to this say I still occasionally have the dream where I am dying and wish I could turn the clock back. I think I will always have this dream from time to time as it has been such a major part of my life.

The day dawned when I was due to go back to work. It had been agreed I could go in for half days and if it got too much I could go home even earlier than that. I wouldn't be secretary I would be word processor operator. Annette came to collect me in her car. Words can't sum up how I was feeling. I was shaking with fear. But I had to try for Mum, Dad and Stu.

The journey from my house to the Town Hall seemed to take forever. The walk from her car to my office was like an eternity. I didn't see many people I knew and to be honest some were ok and some weren't. The ones that were ok didn't say didn't say much just "hi" or "how are you" the usual stuff and they went on their way. It was a world away from the previous months. Then if Mum had dragged me to the town and I happened to see any Town Hall staff some, not all, would actually cross the road to avoid me. But now because I was back at work they thought I was ok and one of them again.

Once I was installed at my work station and a word processor was in front of me I felt a bit safer.

POLES APART

I could just type and loose myself in it. I didn't even drink anything so I wouldn't have to go to the toilet and see anybody. As the time approached for me to go home I began to panic. Nobody was aware of it. I had booked a taxi to take me home. The girls in my office were all friendly and really good with me. Julia, who I have mentioned previously, was a full time temporary typist, one of the members of staff brought in to cover my absence. As time went on she would become a very good friend of mine.

I left the office and prayed I wouldn't see many people. I concentrated on my breathing, taking deep breaths and thinking not long now and I'll be safe at home. I still wasn't taking my medication as I didn't see how it would work if I was dying.

Once I was in the taxi I felt safe. Mum had gone back to work sometime before but I didn't mind. When I got home I felt safe again. As soon as Mum and Dad came home from work that day they said they were so proud of me. Dad said "Each day it'll get easier Shell".

It was so true by taking little steps I was eventually able to take bigger ones. At work it was a nine minute wonder me coming back. I was an object of interest at first but life moves on and before long it was as if I'd never been away.

One of the first big steps was to have a night out. Sandra, one of my friends from the Dolphin Centre (who I would like to say was a good friend whilst I was ill). She would phone me and visit me. She suggested a girl's night out on the town. Another friend from the Dolphin, Linda was also a good friend. I agreed to go.

I was in a terrible state before hand but a couple of days before the night out I made myself go into a clothes shop on my own and get a new outfit. All my old "going out" clothes didn't fit me (the old perfect slim, immaculate Michelle was long gone). By this stage I had also started getting the bus and not taxis, another big step.

The day of the night out dawned. It was a Saturday. I spent a long time getting ready. I had a nice relaxing bath. I played some of my relaxing therapy music and just tried to calm my nerves. I made up my face to the best of my ability and put on my new outfit. Nobody looking at me who didn't know me could possibly imagine what was going on inside me (I truly believe you should never judge people you don't know. I have heard bitchy girls saying upon seeing a very attractive girl "Who does she think she is – she loves herself". How can they say that? That girl could have all sorts of traumas going on in her life. Usually going people who are fat, lazy or have no get up and go or willpower says these things. Instead of trying to change their lives for the better, they just sit and wallow in self pity and begrudge anybody trying to make the most out of their own lives – "Self pity is no pity").

POLES APART

I walked round to Sandra's house. She lived on her own in a house about ten minutes walk away. This was another big step.

For three years while I was going out with Phil I hardly ever went on girl's nights out. I was so wrapped up with Phil – he was my life. I kept in touch with Angie but she was settled with Ian and didn't go out much. Claire lived in London and I only saw her occasionally. Although I liked some of the girls I worked with I didn't have much in common with them and didn't see them socially.

We got the bus into town and met some of Sandra's friends. Some of them knew I'd been ill and some didn't – they were all friendly. I began to relax and enjoy myself. I clearly remember being in "Humphreys" a popular public house which at the time played 70s cheesy music. We were all dancing to a song from "Greece" the movie and I suddenly thought I've missed out on this. After all we were just having fun with your friends. Since I was eighteen I had been in two relationships with hardly any break in between. I had quite a few drinks and for one night I could forget my troubles and have a good time.

At the end of the night, as pre-arranged, I stayed at Sandra's house. We lay in bed giggling and gossiping about the night out. After she had fallen asleep I lay in the darkness thinking if I knew I wasn't dying and could start over I'd like to live with Sandra and start having fun like young girls are supposed to (I was still only 22!).

I went home next morning feeling down. It was great while it lasted my fairytale night out. But in the cold light of day I still couldn't shake off my fear that I was dying and there was no point making long-term plans.

Some weeks passed by, Work was definitely getting easier to go to. Some days I even found myself looking forward to it! I had had a couple more nights out. I had a night out with Annette, Julia and Julia's wonderful husband Eddie (Julia and Eddie would become good friends to me and Billy in the future).

One night I went to bed and had a really vivid dream. Something in the dream was telling me to start over again. Of course I wasn't dying. If I was I would have had some symptoms by now i.e. pains etc. The tablets and stardrops hadn't done any harm and by taking small steps I was well on the way to making a full recovery.

Upon waking I remembered the dream immediately and every detail of it. I lay in bed (it was a Sunday) and made a life changing decision. Today is the first day of the rest of my life. I am not dying, it stuck me that if I was dying I would be feeling ill by now (it was about five months since my breakdown). I felt really healthy. When I got up I felt as if a weight had been lifted from my shoulders. I felt joy and actually looked forward to the day ahead. I didn't discuss my dream with anyone.

From that day I seemed to regain my "Joy de vivre" and I fell in love with life again. I looked forward to what each day would bring. I was going out more and more and having such a good time. I had gone back to work full-time and was enjoying my job (before I got ill I always enjoyed my job because I had worked so hard to get it and to get on at the Town Hall and I knew I was good at it).

I was still going to Richmond for my therapy once a week. She said I was "wearing too many hats and trying to please everyone". She said I should please myself more and make myself happy. So that is what I set out to do.

One morning upon waking I looked around my bedroom and realised there was one thing holding me back – this room. I was happy but felt I would be happier leaving home and starting afresh away from all the bad memories my bedroom held.

I told Mum and Dad of my plans to leave home. They were apprehensive but when I told them my reasons they couldn't stop me.

I decided to ask Sandra if she wanted a lodger. She said it might spoil our friendship. I wasn't disheartened. I decided to look for a flat.

The Enforcement Officer at work, Kevin, was renting his house out – he had moved in with his girlfriend. I asked him if I could be his tenant. He agreed.

I felt so happy. I couldn't wait to move into the house. My head was full of plans. I was forever making lists of things I needed to do and things I needed to buy.

My car was on its last legs. It was quite old and Phil and I had run it into the ground. One day I broke down in it. Instead of getting it fixed, on impulse, I went out and bought another. I left my car where it had broken down and didn't get it towed away for three days. I didn't care – nothing could dent my happiness.

The day arrived for me to move in. I had bought all new things for the house, apart from furniture. I got a bank loan – what the hell I thought its only money (I'm alive who cares). Me, my family and friends spent all day cleaning and getting it nice. I went out that night and had a fabulous time. The old Michelle had returned with a vengeance. I was more bubbly, confident and outgoing than ever. I was still overweight but I didn't care. I had bought new clothes and I still made the best of myself by doing my hair and make-up.

POLES APART

At the end of the night I returned home alone. I sat down in the living room and looked around. I just felt on top of the world.

I went to bed and slept like a baby. I woke up early, at about six in the morning. It was summer by then and light was flooding through the bedroom curtains. I didn't feel tired. I felt so full of happiness and energy. I couldn't lie in bed wasting the morning I wanted to get up and do things.

I got up and made myself a cup of tea. While the kettle was boiling I noticed the kitchen windows were dirty. Well I would start by cleaning the windows I thought. I didn't have any windowlene or other window cleaning products but that didn't stop me. I just got a bucket of hot soapy water and began to clean them. The sun was shining through the windows and the joy I was feeling was immense – anything was possible I told myself.

I seemed to have acquired a "devil may care" attitude to everything. I put walls around me so nobody could get in and dent my happiness. Every mad, impulsive crazy thing I did I justified in my own head by thinking well I played the slim, perfect girlfriend, the hard worker, the good friend, the loving daughter and look where it got me. Now it's all about me – I'll do what I want and when I want to do it. I never hurt anybody intentionally because that is just not in my nature.

Now I know I suffer from bi-polar syndrome I realise I was still ill only the scales had tipped. So instead of being very low I was very high. When we look back my parents, especially Mum, refers to it as my "mad phase". Of course they didn't understand bi-polar and were still worried about me thinking I had gone off the rails, which I had to a degree.

I was always going out. If my friends couldn't make it I would go out on my own. I was so confident I didn't care. I made loads of friends – I would talk to anyone.

People with bi-polar have a high sex drive, this can take effect especially when on a "high". Luckily, I didn't go too mad although I did have a few one night stands. This was so out of character for me because when I met Phil we waited for weeks before we became lovers.

I would have parties at the drop of a hat and loved nothing more than a houseful of people having a great time. I do remember one party and Sandra and Linda my friends asking to see me alone in my bedroom. "We're worried about you Shell" they said "What's there to be worried about? I'm doing great – I'm really happy" I said. Looking back of course they would have been worried about me because I had changed so much. I seem to remember getting angry with them because I thought they didn't think I deserved to be happy, especially after everything I had gone through.

As I have said before, I was never nasty but if anybody tried to calm me down, or told me to take things easy, or not make rash decisions, I wouldn't listen and I just blocked them out. They can go to hell I thought. I don't care. It's my life – the life I didn't think I was going to have.

I have always loved animals and I went to the Cats Protection League and got myself two kittens – I called them Brandy and Coke.

Mum and Dad had decided to go on holiday to Greece. They asked me if I wanted to go with them. I would have preferred to go with my friends but none of them could afford it.

A couple of weeks before we were due to go I was shopping in Middlesbrough with my good friend Sue. I saw a tattoo shop and on impulse I went and got one. My Mum was horrified. I had also started to have a cigarette when I was having a drink. I didn't smoke during the day only at night. All these things shocked Mum and Dad. I had always been such a goody two shoes (the whole five years at Long field I never got into trouble, never forgot my homework, always tried my best (my reports were always very good) and eventually I became a Prefect.

Unbeknown to them I had also started to dabble in soft drugs. Just a bit of pot now and then. I tried speed once or twice but it did nothing for me. Looking back it was no wonder as I was high as a kite with my illness.

Before we flew to Crete we stayed the weekend with our relatives in Oldham near Manchester. I have a half cousin called Dianne and on our first night in Oldham I went out with Dianne and her friends. We had a ball. One of Dianne's male friends (I can't remember his name) was house sitting for the weekend at his sisters luxury house. They had their own business and were very rich. He suggested we all went back and carried on the party.

We arrived at the house in a suburb of Manchester – it was amazing. It had an indoor swimming pool, pool room, fully stocked bar, 2 Jacuzzis. I rang Mum and Dad who were staying at my aunties to say I was staying the night and we all stayed the weekend. What a weekend!

On the Monday morning I went to my Aunties to get changed and get my things for the holiday. When we arrived at the airport I went mad buying all sorts in the duty free. My spending had gone haywire.

We arrived at our resort in Crete in the early hours of the morning. We had a drink and then we were shown to our studio. It was tiny. It was going to be impossible for the three of us to share this small studio for two weeks.

The next day when the rep arrived Dad explained our predicament. He said we would pay extra if they would find me another room. The best she could do was an apartment of my own at the far side of the resort. This worked to everyone's advantage. I was out of their hair, they could get a bit of peace and I got my freedom.

My apartment had two bedrooms, bathroom, open plan kitchen, dining and living room. It was on the ground floor of a two storey building, facing the main road. I used to love nothing better than to have a shower after a days sunbathing, pour myself a drink and sit by the patio watching the world go by.

I had only been there a couple of days when I realised I didn't have much money left. When I told Dad he wasn't happy but he agreed to loan me some and I would pay him back when I got home. Only he said he wouldn't give me it all at once. I had to go and see him every day to get my allowance for the day.

My days took on a routine pattern. I would get up at leisure (depending on how late I had went to bed!), walk to Mum and Dad's apartment. Usually I would find them sunbathing. Have a chat and maybe a drink with them. Get my money and walk to the beach near my apartment. There was a really good beach bar there and I would find a lounger, claim it with my towel. Then I would alternate between sunbathing and sitting at the bar chatting and having a drink. I had got to know all the barmen and waitresses by now and some other holidaymakers.

One day whilst I was at the beach a stray dog took a fancy to me. I love dogs, so I made a fuss of it. When I bought a sandwich for my lunch and set about eating it on my lounger, it looked at me with big soulful hungry eyes. Of course the dog ended up having half of the sandwich! As the afternoon progressed it would wander off from time to time but after a short while would re-appear and lie at my side by the sun lounger.

When I packed up my things to go at the end of the afternoon it followed me all the way to my apartment. I thought when I went inside that it would just go on its way. How wrong was I?

That evening when I was all dressed and on my way out I found it laid by the front door. As most of the bars were open taverns, it just waited outside for me at each one I visited that night.

By this stage I had made friends with an English girl who had been let down by her friends and was holidaying alone. She thought it was hilarious that the dog was following me everywhere. It ended up staying at my apartment with me the whole holiday and constantly stayed by my side (I just had to make sure we were both out when the maid visited).

I had a really fabulous holiday and made loads of friends. Towards the end of the holidays I asked Mum and Dad round to my apartment to say thanks by way of a meal and a drink. I decided to do a pasta dish and went shopping for the ingredients. I got ham to go in the tomato/veg sauce. The dog looked so longingly at the ham I ended up giving most of it to him. Eventually when they were eating it Mum commented "By there's not much meat in this Shell!"

Before the end of the holiday a friend I had made, who worked in one of the local taverns, asked if I wanted a job and I could share her apartment. She had been a printer in the south of England somewhere and had found it stressful. So one day she handed her notice in and landed up in Crete. She found the job and apartment and loved her new life. I was sorely tempted but Mum and Dad reminded me of everything I would loose – my wonderful job at the Town Hall (the one that had already contributed towards my two breakdowns!) As I have previously said, my parents were wonderful but they don't understand office stress. It is only years later when I talk about conditions at the Town Hall that they understand. At the time I just got on with it – I didn't know any different. Mum had always worked in bars, shops or factories. Dad had always worked in factories. They did not have any office experience. The admin section I worked in was so disorganized.   I am not bitter but some days I get frustrated when I look back, all I was guilty of was working too hard and I was tret terribly. There are plenty of staff still there doing a lousy job, as little as possible and getting away with it.   People who don't now the way local council's work will find this a bit bar fetched but it is true.

My Projects and Administration Manager and Office Manager weren't horrible people they were quite nice men really just weak men and they let the other managers walk all over them. Consequently, if we went to them with our problems they tried, but rarely sorted them out.

I was working for a Director and three section heads. Each was in competition with each other in the cut-throat world of Local Government. They didn't care how much they were dumping on me as long as the job got done and their work was complete and they got their "brownie points". As I said to Mum and Dad, in a factory, pub or shop you do one thing at a time. You wouldn't be expected to serve two people at once would you?

As we left the resort on our last day and headed to the airport by coach I started to cry "What's wrong Shell?" Mum said. I explained that I had seen my stray dog sitting at the edge of the pavement. "Only you could cry for a dog, most girls cry after broken holiday romances not you!"

POLES APART

When we arrived home in Darlington I went to the bank to get the money to pay Dad back. I was shocked when I noticed how overdrawn I was. But I wasn't going to worry. I put it to the back of my mind.

Money was getting to be a bit of a problem. Kevin, my landlord's cheque had bounced and I had bills to pay. I decided to look for a part-time bar job (I had never returned to the Dolphin Centre).

I got a couple of nights a week in Perry's, a trendy pub in Darlington. I worked there for a couple of weeks but one Friday night before I was due to start work I popped into the "Green Dragon" a pub I had started frequenting. I liked it in the Dragon and I knew quite a few people. Susan's boyfriend, Mark, was there with his friends. We were having a good time. I thought "What the hell I can't be bothered going to work". I got someone to ring in sick for me. |Unluckily for me I was spotted rolling out of the pub later that night by someone from Perry's who told the Manager – that was the end of me at Perry's!

As I mentioned previously, I had started to have the odd joint. One Saturday night I had been out and met a friend called Simon. At the end of the evening he came back to mine for a drink and to "skin up". He stayed the night on the sofa. He was just a friend. Next morning he disappeared.

When he returned a bit later he said he had someone he wanted me to meet – his friend Joe. He was from Liverpool and we got on like a house on fire. It wasn't love at first sight more like lust!

All three of us went round to his house. Jo made us some food. He was a great cook. Afterwards we went for a drive and ended up picking magic mushrooms. Joe knew a spot where he went regularly. When we got back to Joes we sat around for the rest of the afternoon drinking magic mushroom tea. Joe put on this "trippy" music and we were all off our heads. I had never met anyone like Joe – he seemed as happy, free and outgoing as I was now – I thought I had met my soul mate!

I stayed the night at his place and he woke me up in the early hours of the morning and proposed to me. It was crazy but I accepted. As soon as it was light we were going to go to Gretna Green and get married. I rang the Town Hall and asked for a couple of day's holiday – at this stage I didn't say why.

When we arrived at Gretna we were told you had to do the Banns and book etc, so we couldn't get married. The crazy thing was we agreed to tell people we were married anyway. We got a cheap gold ring and told everyone we were married!

We started living together and I collected my kittens and the things I needed from my rented house. I did leave the house in a bit of a state, but when I moved in it was really dingy and I had decorated it and tidied it up so I thought this evened the score. Kev and I fell out for ages after this but I wouldn't let it bother me.

Jo was a DJ in a local nightclub and he knew some shady characters. We had lots of parties but everyone only smoked blow or had magic mushrooms and I thought they were sound.

We had been living together for a few weeks when things began to change. Looking back I was the one who was changing. From being "super high" where I didn't care about anything, I came down a bit. I was still happy but I started to see things more clearly.

It was Autumn/Winter and I am never as happy in winter as summer. I don't suffer from SAD as I don't feel depressed in winter but I definitely feel much more alive in Spring/Summer.

Certain things Jo did started getting on my nerves and the way we were living. We started to argue a lot and one night we had a major bust up. I moved into the spare room and next day we decided we would be better as friends sharing the house as we wanted different things.

Things came to a head one night. I was asleep in bed and I heard a great thud followed by lots of footsteps. It was the door being kicked down by the drugs squad. They searched the house from top to bottom and I was in a state. They didn't find anything but I felt as if I'd been banged on the head which finally made me see what I was doing with my life.

As quickly as I could I got some essentials together and walked out of the door and never looked back (I didn't take the kittens at this stage I got them later).

I didn't want to go to Mum and Dad. The thought of living at home again filled me with fear – the house held too many bad memories. I went to Sue's. Sue and I had been friends since I worked with her in Environmental Health when I was sixteen. She is two years older than me and two more different people you could wish to meet. But we just gelled – they say opposites attract.

Sue was engaged when we first met and living with her boyfriend and his parents and seemed more mature and worldly than me. A lot of people think Sue is hard-faced but I detected warmth in her. Sue is as "straight as a die". She will never stab you in the back. Sue speaks her mind but wouldn't intentionally hurt anyone. In the two-faced world of the Town Hall people don't always like her but give me one of Sue any day to ten of the back-stabbers. We had been out socially once or twice but at that stage weren't the firm friends we would later become, when her boyfriend Dave cheated on her. The relationship was over and his mother kicked Sue out onto the street. Sue didn't have any parents to turn to. A friend took her in but their house was already full to the rafters. I felt sorry for her. She was looking around for a bedsit but they were all grotty. I told Mum and Dad about her and asked if she could come and live with us and share my bedroom while she sorted herself out. They agreed and she came to live with us, initially for about a month, but Mum and Dad let her stay while she sorted out trying to buy her own house. I have every respect for Sue. She had a very hard childhood but she is a trier. She never feels sorry for herself she just gets on with it. She now lives in a fabulous house that her lovely husband Kev built for them. She has two gorgeous boys – Jack and Ben. Yet despite everything that has happened to her (she spent some of her childhood in a Children's Home and was fostered) people say "who does she think she is?" These people make me sick they are so steeped in bitterness. Everything Sue has she deserves because she is a fighter and she won't give up on life. We were good friends until I met Phil and then we just sort of drifted apart. Probably because I was so wrapped up in Phil. When I was ill she would ring me and had showed herself to be a true friend. I had seen a lot of Sue over the summer.

When I arrived at Sue's she said I did the right thing leaving. I was so naïve he could have been dealing drugs or anything and even though I was totally unaware and innocent I could have been dragged down with him. She offered me her couch to sleep on, as she had a lodger Dave (her ex brother in law) staying in her spare room.

Living at Sue's came at the right time. I was still "happy" but under Sue's sensible influence I calmed down a bit. I still did some mad, zany things but that's just me. I wasn't doing anything totally out of character. I had a great time living with Sue, we had some laughs! Also because Sue's had to be, she's very organized with money. By this stage I was in a right mess with money (before I met Phil I had always been really careful, probably down to my childhood, but Phil was reckless with money and believed in living for today, sod tomorrow). His attitude rubbed off on me and with me being high as well I had gone off the deep end with regards money. Sue sorted out all of my finances. She rang all the credit card companies and the bank and re-negotiated amounts that I could manage for each debt. Because I had a full time job I had to pay quite a lot and I didn't have much to live on. I had to start being sensible with money and that has continued to this day.

Stuart my brother was still living with his girlfriend Sandra and I had become friendly with her. About a week before Christmas I had a night out with Sandra and a couple of her friends. We went to a couple of pubs. In about the third/fourth pub we were standing near the bar when Billy, someone I had met once or twice in the Green Dragon, came and started talking to me. When I first saw him in the Dragon I thought he was quite good looking but seemed a bit standoffish, although we didn't speak. But I had talked to him since a couple of times and I really liked him – but I didn't think he was interested in me. As we were talking somebody pushed past me and made a sarcastic remark. Billy said "Don't let anybody put you down – you're lovely the way you are".

I know it sounds corny but Billy make me feel safe. I wouldn't say it was love at first sight (but I never think that lasts) but there was definitely an attraction. But it was more like a slow burning flame that grew and grew into something so strong it could get us through anything!

Billy is a bit like Sue in some ways. He has walls around him and doesn't let many people in. He is a wonderful person when you get to know him but he had to erect these barriers in order to survive his terrible childhood. He was born in Paisley, near Glasgow, Scotland. When he was two and his brother was one his mother had a breakdown. She put his younger brother in a home (Billy has never seen him to this day) and Billy's Granny took Billy in. Billy doesn't go into much detail abut his childhood but from what I can gather it was very tough. His Granny loved him but liked a drink and reading between the lines he "dragged himself up". He didn't always have a lot to eat and didn't attend school much. He used to take the neighbors dogs and disappear into the countryside surrounding Glasgow for days. The dogs killed rabbits and he would gut them, cook them and eat them. Nobody reported him missing. It was another world up there! His Dad rarely bothered with him and when his mother recovered she re-married and had three other children. She just forgot about Billy and his brother – what a total bitch – how could she call herself a mother!

Sandra and her friends said they were going to the next pub – I said I'd catch them up. I never did. We carried on talking until it was last orders! His friends he was out with had gone as well. We started walking to a taxi rank – there were no taxis in sight. Billy said did I want to get a bite to eat and take it back to his house – no funny business! I trusted him and agreed. We walked to his house which was quite near the town centre. He was renting it but I was amazed when we entered. It was spic and span – you could eat your dinner off the living room carpet. Most men living alone would live like slobs – not Billy! Because of his childhood he appreciates what he gets and looks after things and likes a tidy house. I am the total opposite. Although I was very organised at work, at home I am not dirty just messy. At Billy's there was a place for everything and everything in its place. We sat talking for ages and eventually I fell asleep on the sofa. When I woke next morning Billy had put a pillow under my head and covered me with a blanket. He was asleep in the chair. I looked around the room – I felt so at home being there with Billy. He woke not long after. Billy was out of work at the time and didn't have a lot of cash so there wasn't much in to eat, but he still went to the local shop and bought all the ingredients to cook me a big fry-up.

After breakfast I wanted to go home to get changed. I looked out of the window and it had started to snow. Billy lent me his big parker coat (neither of us had enough money left for a taxi) and walked me home.

I asked him when I could give him his coat back. He said I'm going to borrow a couple of quid and I'll be in the Dragon at tea-time. I was so nervous about going to meet him. Because I was falling for him I was worried that he didn't feel the same way. I had been so badly hurt that I was terrified of walking into the pub, him taking the coat and then being cool with me.

My fears were ungrounded – his face lit up when he saw me and after that we were inseparable.

Because a lot of people don't understand Billy (a bit like they don't understand Sue) my family and friends couldn't see what I saw in him at first. My Mum and Dad thought he was just a lay about on the dole willing to sponge off me as I was working. I remember after being with Billy a couple of months, Stephen, my boss, (by then I was Secretary again) saying to Julia "What does Michelle see in Billy?" (Even though he had never met him). In Stephen's eyes, as Billy wasn't working and not living in a posh house or driving a posh car, he was a nothing. As I have said previously, I grew to like Stephen but he was very materialistic and after everything that had happened to me I certainly wasn't. Julia told me that she told Stephen that, in her eyes, Billy gave me stability – which I desperately needed – and loved me for what I was, not some perfect image he was going to mould me into. When I met him I was about three stone overweight. But he said he didn't care it was my pretty face and personality that he had fallen for. He wasn't interested in my money because he knew I was deeply in debt.

You should never judge a book by its cover as just because Billy didn't have any qualifications and had never had a "good" job (he was just temporarily out of work he had been working up until a couple of months before Christmas) he is very intelligent. He is a self-taught man and he amazes me with his general knowledge. When I met him he had just started an Open University course in Music and the Arts but he didn't finish it. He said he wished he had met me earlier because I would have encouraged him to finish it. He is extremely interested in music and he has a very wide and knowledgeable taste. Just because he used to be a biker and has a few tattoos, some snobby people would pigeonhole him and say "thick yob". As I have already said, people like this make me sick. I believe that there is good and bad in all classes and in all walks of life. We all come into the world with nothing and we all go

POLES APART

out with nothing. The person you are and values you have are what matter, not how much money you have. Some of the richest people in the world are the greediest and some of the most poor would share their last bowl of rice – that makes them the better person.

Brian, Billy's best friend and his lovely girlfriend Bev (who isn't with Brian now) always used to reminisce about when I had only been seeing Billy about a week. It was sometime between the Christmas/New Year holiday. I was going out with Sue and a couple of her friends. We all agreed to go in fancy dress. Dave, Sue's lodger was an ex punk so he did my hair and make-up punk style and I wore boxer shorts, a vest and put a bin bag on – what a state I must have looked. Sue came home from work (I had a day's holiday) and said everyone had changed their minds about going in fancy dress. But instead of taking off the punk make-up or getting changed, I thought sod it I'll go out like this. Anybody who truly knows me will know that I like to have a laugh and can laugh at myself. Well when we walked into the Green Dragon later that night Billy's friends were gob-smacked. They thought I was crazy but Billy thought it was funny.

Gradually with living at Sue's and dating Billy I found myself again. Because I was in so much debt and Billy wasn't working we didn't have much cash to go out but we were happy doing simple things. I hate housework but I love to cook. Some nights I would finish work, tell Billy what to buy then I would cook it for us. We would snuggle up on the bed settee in his living room and watch TV/listen to music. Through Billy I acquired a taste for red wine and money permitting we would share a bottle. I had never walked much before I met Billy or taken much interest in the countryside. But he loved nothing better than to go walking. I began to go with him and really enjoyed it. I started to loose some weight and I felt really healthy.

We had been seeing each other a couple of months when he asked me to move in with him. I followed my instincts and agreed. I know people probably think we rushed things but I knew instinctively that Billy was the one for me. We didn't have a lot of material possessions (we didn't have a bed – we slept on the bed settee and didn't even have a hoover – Billy used to get on his hands and knees and brush the carpet with a dustpan and brush (but the important thing was that we had each other).

I remember making a meal for Billy's friend Paul and his wife Jo and we didn't even have four knives and forks we had to borrow from our next door neighbors.

Not long after moving I began to feel physically unwell. I was feeling really tired, my breasts hurt and I started to feel nauseous. I couldn't be pregnant I told myself I was on the pill. I went to the Doctor but she asked me to do a pregnancy test. Of course the devastating thing was that I was. It couldn't have come at a worst possible time in my life. Billy was brilliant with me and said he would stand by me no matter what. My head was in turmoil. Part of me would have liked a baby but the realist side of me knew that I wasn't totally mentally stable yet. I had just got over my breakdown and this would tip me over the edge again. The only other person I told was Sue – she agreed with me. I couldn't tell Angie. She and Ian had just had Travis and they were both totally in love with their bundle of joy. I didn't think they would understand. Dr. Young and the consultant at the hospital were also marvelous. Because of my history of mental illness there was no pressure put on me to keep the baby. After I had made my decision to have a termination, they even agreed that a termination would be best for me. This is the hardest thing I have ever had to do. I just hoped god would forgive me as I had to do it for my own sanity.

Afterwards I got on with my life and tried to push it to the back of my mind. Even now after I have had my two girls I know I couldn't have coped back then.

This knocked me back a bit but I don't think people were aware of any change in me. I put my mask on for the outside world. Billy reassured me we had made the right decision when I felt a bit low.

Months went by and I felt stronger.

When Billy had been twenty-two his girlfriend at the time Fran had a daughter to Billy. They called her Natalie. They broke up when Natalie was about four. When I got with Billy Natalie was eleven. She was a beautiful young girl and she had a nice nature. I took to her straight away and she spent some weekends with us. Billy always says it is how I was with Natalie when I first met her that clenched it for him. One of his previous girlfriends had been jealous of Natalie. How could anybody be jealous of a child – she was a part of Billy and I loved her. She went through a rebellious teenager state but deep down she is a good person. Billy was working by then and we were better of financially and started to get things for the house. His friend Tony had bought a taxi and we were in partnership. One of the first things we bought was a double bed. It was sheer luxury after sleeping for months on a bed settee with springs sticking up your bum.

We had some weekends away. We went to visit a friend of Billy's who had moved to Loch Lomand in Scotland. That was to be the start of my love affair with the Scottish West Highlands. It is me and Billy's favorite place to visit in the whole of the British Isles. I especially love to visit in autumn. It is so beautiful with all the rich colors. When I look up at the majestic mountains and the lochs nestled at their feet a feeling of peace and tranquility washes over me.

My and Billy got ourselves a dog. We couldn't afford to buy one so we scoured the papers and shop windows for any "free to good home" adverts. We eventually found our darling little Roxy. She was a cross-breed puppy and was supposed to be half German shepherd. Even when she was fully grown she was only little and Billy said I used to treat her like a baby. She loved nothing better than to sit on my knee while I watched TV and get petted.

Time went by. As anybody with any sense will tell you a relationship has to be worked at. We did argue and fall out sometimes but we always made up and worked at our relationship. I know my messiness drives Billy mad and sometimes he thinks I have "verbal diorea". But I also think Billy can be hot-headed and loose his temper easily. But everyone has their faults and we loved each other.

Everything was fine at work, but was still hectic and busy most of the time. The whole of my eleven years at the Town Hall I never had a "cushy office job". I wish I had then maybe I wouldn't have had three breakdowns!

By now the management had realised how much work there was and the temps were still there. Originally before I was ill there was Elaine (part-time Secretary), me (part-time Secretary and part-time Word Processor Operator), Annette (full-time Word Processor Operator) and Gwen (part-time Word Processor Operator) = three full-time positions. Now there was all the above with the addition of Julia (full-time Word Processor Operator) and Maureen (part-time Word Processor Operator). Before I was ill it doesn't take a genius to work out who was doing their own work plus the work of one and a half others!

As Julia was experienced and older and spoke her mind, she let it be known to those at fault that she blamed them for putting so much work and pressure on someone so young as to make them ill. She always said because I was so efficient at my job they had taken advantage of my good nature and just dumped on me without thinking or caring!

One day in late summer when I was twenty-five. I and Billy had gone to Scarborough with Natalie. We had a lovely day and we were sitting on the sand soaking up the sun when Billy said he was going to get a surprise for me. Natalie went with him and when they returned he got down on one knee and proposed to me. He had got a "cubic cigona" ring I had admired in a shop earlier. Of course I said yes and I was really happy (later when we had more money he would replace it with a diamond one but I still wear that ring on my other hand – it has sentimental value).

POLES APART

We set about organizing our wedding. The taxi business at the time was very haphazard and Billy's earnings were very up and down. A lot depended on luck and we didn't have much of that with regards money. I was still paying my debts and things weren't as bad as they had been. We would have loved to have bought our house but I was blacklisted after getting into all my debt.

My lovely parents and Nanna and Grandad helped us out a bit and the date was set for the tenth of June in the following year. I was having a traditional while wedding. With me being the only girl I knew it would mean a lot to Dad to walk me up the aisle.

From setting the date to our wedding day our luck with money seemed to get even worse. If a taxi is "off the road" i.e. needing repairs etc you still have to pay radio rent to the taxi company. One day about a month before Christmas a motorcyclist crashed into Billy. It was the motorcyclist's fault but he had no insurance! Our taxi was off the road for a couple of weeks and we were in dire straits.

I'll always remember that Christmas. We couldn't afford gifts for anybody or each other but our family understood. We couldn't afford a tree or decorations for the house but this didn't get us down. Luckily we were going to Mums for dinner so we didn't have to worry about food and what always gets us by when times are hard is to remember the important things in life. Sadly, things many people forget in this materialistic age. We were both fairly young, healthy, had each other and the love of a good family and true friends. If you have these things you are truly blessed. You have to be optimistic and look to the future when things will get better. I remember getting up before Billy that Christmas morning and sitting by the fire with a mug of tea. I remember feeling happy and at peace with myself. Nothing could ever be as bad as the Christmas before my breakdown (when you've been in hell nothing could ever be as bad!)

Financially things didn't improve drastically after Christmas and about two months before the wedding Billy decided to look for another job. He got a job in a factory where my Dad worked. The money was poor but at least we knew how much was coming in each week and where we stood.

I had started to get a bit panicky about how we were going to pay for the wedding but luckily my Nanna borrowed us the money we needed so my mind could be at rest.

The night before my wedding day I stayed at Mum and Dads. This was the first time I had stayed in my old room since leaving home. Sue came round and we had a lovely girly night. We had a drink and she did my eyebrows and nails. Mum and Dad were out with my relatives who had come up for the wedding. Sue left before they came in, she was going to be my Chief Bridesmaid and she wanted an early night. I went to bed in my old room. I remember lying in bed and thinking how far I'd come since I was last sleeping in that room. I felt true happiness and now I had changed and met Billy I couldn't get ill again.

When Dad saw me on my wedding day there were tears in his eyes. "I'm so proud of you Shell, not many girls your age have gone through what you've gone through and look at you now" I had to blink to stop myself from crying and ruining my make-up. I had a fabulous day and loved feeling like a princess in my gorgeous wedding dress.

We went to Majorca for our honeymoon on a late deal package holiday. We had a fabulous time and I was on a "high". Like I have said before I didn't at this stage in my life know I suffered from bi-polar. Because I was with Billy and he has a calming influence on me I didn't go too high but I was quite reckless with money. We didn't have much spending money and I bought three pairs of shoes! On the last day we didn't even have enough money left to buy bottled water!

The memory that stands out the best from that wonderful honeymoon was when Billy sang to me. He is a very good singer and we were in a Karaoke bar one night. He told the Compare it was our honeymoon and he sang "Volare" by Dean Martin to me. I love Dean Martin's songs they are so romantic. The audience went mad clapping afterwards. When we came home I was still high for a few weeks but gradually I came down.

I was friendly with some of Billy's friend's wives/girlfriends. I used to have the occasional night out with them. They had organized a day trip to Blackpool in the October and I had agreed to go. When I had agreed to go in the Summer I was still on a high but by the time the trip came round I was feeling a bit run-down. Now I know I suffer from bi-polar I was slightly depressed (not deeply). I had been high all summer and with short days and cold depressing weather I wasn't feeling myself. Things were fine at work and Billy and I were ok and I wasn't worried about money but bi-polar is an illness and the scales had tipped again.

Now I know all the signs I realise I was depressed. Not severely depressed or psychotic like I had been in the past. I could have slept the clock round I was always tired. I was eating too much. I had put about a stone on. (By this stage in my life I was slim again). Once I got with Billy and I was walking a lot and eating sensibly the weight came off and I felt better for it.

When the day came to go to Blackpool I was dreading it. It was an effort getting through the day and I kept thinking of Billy back at home and wishing I could be with him. I wasn't as bubbly as usual and the girls noticed but I said I thought I was a bit run-down.

When I look back I wasn't myself all winter but when you've been severely depressed/psychotic nothing is ever as bad as that. There was just the usual pressure at work and it wasn't getting me down. I know as long as I am sleeping I am ok – which I was. Billy wasn't really aware because I was still me just not as bubbly as usual.

Whilst I had been "high" in the summer some of the girls had suggested a girly week in Bennidorm for the following summer. This sounded like a great idea and I agreed to go. In the middle of the winter I started to dread it but once spring came round I started to feel better and began to look forward to my holiday with the girls. Money was just as tight as ever so I got a couple of evenings bar work, working in a Working Men's Club to pay for my holiday.

About a month before I was due to go to Bennidorm I was at work. I was at my desk (I was Word Processor Operator that day) typing a letter when I overheard two of the Planning Officers discussing an article in that day's paper (it might have been front page news). They were in the next room but the door between the two offices was open. I suddenly sat bolt upright. They were talking about a man who had been a Social Worker, who had been awarded a massive payout for having to handle too much stress at work which eventually lead to two breakdowns. I couldn't wait to get my hands on that newspaper and read the article.

When eventually I got hold of the paper and read it, it was like a revelation. The man could have been me! Julia was still working with me and when she read it she said I think you have a good case for compensation for what you went through.

For the rest of the day I frantically typed away on my Word Processor. To all the other members of staff I just looked like I was working but no I was stating my claim against the Council and putting down all the facts of what had happened to me. As I was older and wiser I knew wholeheartedly that what happened to me was solely down to stress. I had been in a happy relationship at the time of my breakdown. I had a loving family, no money worries – no it was just severe stress at work that had tipped me over the edge and nearly made me loose everything, my life included. I wanted some heads to roll and somebody to finally acknowledge what they had done to me.

That evening I couldn't wait to get home to Billy to tell him. He was totally behind me, as likewise were Mum and Dad. All that weekend I was on a high and I couldn't wait to get to work on the Monday morning to see someone from the Union.

The Union thought I had a good case and sent my documentation away to the Union solicitors to get an opinion. I knew it would be a while before I heard anything so I just got on with my life.

I was so happy because I felt that at last the last piece of the jigsaw had slotted into place. I was truly happy with Billy but there was a tiny niggly feeling at the back of my mind about ever getting that stressed at work (like I have said previously once you've had a breakdown you never forget). Now I knew they wouldn't be able to make me ill again – or if they did heads would roll and they'd pay for it.

The holiday to Bennidorm came round. We had a great time and I was on a high.

When we came home I and Billy started rowing a lot. I was quite selfish and wanted to go out with the girls all the time. He had never minded me having nights out with my friends (he wasn't the jealous type) but I was taking advantage.

One day there was a letter waiting for me when I got home from work. It was from the Union Solicitors. They admitted I had been under a lot of stress but didn't think that I would win my case. I felt crushed. But I was determined not to let it get me down. I sat down and thought about all the good things in my life and how far I'd come since my second breakdown. I also realised how awful I'd been to Billy and we found each other again.

By this time Billy was working for the same company as Julia's husband Eddie.

Everything was ok at work. Until one day I had been on my lunch and when Helen, a Word Processor Operator who had replaced Annette, had gone for lunch, Julia asked to have a word with me. I couldn't believe what she had to say. Apparently, whilst I had been at lunch Helen had had a "fit". She had ranted and raved about hating me that much that she was going to "punch my lights out one of these days". I was in shock! Helen was a bit of a strange girl. She was very quiet at work and wouldn't say boo to a goose. She always seemed very nervy. Even though I didn't have much in common with her I was always nice to her. It is not in my nature to be nasty to anyone (that is one of my problems because by doing this people hurt me). Julia was also shocked that it had happened as she couldn't understand where she was coming from. Julia had thought she had better warn me to be on my guard with her. I wished Julia hadn't said anything because it chewed away at me. "Why didn't she like me, what had I done to her?" I kept asking myself. When I told Billy that evening he said "Forget it some people are bitches and she sounds like one, she's probably jealous of you because you're bubbly and she just sits in the corner" (I knew she had a lot of personal troubles in her life). Billy is so strong and never lets anybody take advantage of him but sadly I'm not like that – I wish I was!

POLES APART

After that I went out of my way to be really nice to her and she totally took advantage. I would say she started to bully me in a small way. If I said one thing she would say the other, wait for me to retaliate and when I didn't she knew she had won. She would say she would be back for dinner at a certain time and when she wasn't and came in a bit later I never said anything even though I got less time for my dinner.

I told my fears to Elaine but she said she liked Helen. Since I had come back to work from my last breakdown Julia said I carried Elaine. When she was at work I was always in the next room to help her and sort out any queries out but when I was Secretary it was her days off and I had to cope on my own. No wonder Elaine liked Helen. I later found out that she had been telling lies to Elaine about what we were saying behind her back. Who did Elaine believe? The person who had enabled her to keep her job by carrying her or the bitch Helen who had been there two minutes – of course she believed Helen. I was so hurt after everything I had done for Elaine. But as the saying goes "You just need one bad apple to rot the barrel".

We had always got on in our small office. We were all different but never argued. By this stage Annette had left. There was Julia (full-time Senior Typist), me (part-time Secretary, part-time Word Processor Operator), Elaine (part-time Secretary),

Helen (full-time Word Processor Operator), Gwen (part-time Word Processor Operator) and Maureen (part-time Word Processor Operator). Up until this point Julia and Helen had always got on but Julia became wary of her.

A few weeks went by. Then Helen started being funny with Julia. Julia and I decided to go and see Ray (our Admin and Projects Manager). We thought that if he knew of the scenario and she ever did totally flip in the office he would have been forewarned. He said there had been some trouble with her in her previous department and he would keep an eye on the situation.

Our friends Lisa and Simon had put their house on the market. Billy and I had always liked it. It was a three bedroomed end terraced house with garage near the South Park in Darlington. It was an unusual shape and quite roomy and the way it was positioned meant that lots of sunlight got in and it wasn't dingy like our house could be sometimes. As it had been over five years since I had got myself in the financial mess and I was near to paying most of my debts off, we decided to see if we could get a mortgage. We were introduced to a Financial Advisor through Simon and Lisa and he sorted one out for us. We were overjoyed that we were getting our own home. The mortgage wasn't much more than the rent we were paying.

POLES APART

Although the scenario at work with Helen still chewed me a bit I pushed it to the back of my mind and concentrated on making plans for our house.

We were due to complete in early September. Sue and Kev were getting married in August and I was going to be Matron of Honor. I had been looking forward to it for months.

A couple of weeks before Sue's wedding the contract Billy was working on came to an end. He would be needed on the next job but we didn't know when it would start. I started to fret about money. It seemed we were taking a big step in buying the house as Billy's job was so up and down. Luckily I was the main breadwinner and we could just about manage on my wages.

By this time in my life I was sick of being taken for a mug at work. Julia was always saying I was the backbone of our section, who were involved in some major projects i.e. revamping of the Market Square, Shopmobility, and Major's Design Awards. Increasingly, I felt I was doing more and more work. One day I'd just had enough and I asked if I could speak to Stephen in private. He agreed that I was taking on more and more responsibility and he relied on me. He asked how I would feel about becoming his full-time PA. Elaine would be a part-time PA and do more hours as required.

I thought that Elaine would be pleased with this. In all the years since she had first went part-time she had showed no inclination to go full-time again, even though her daughter was at school now. She pretended she was pleased but I could tell her nose was pushed out of joint. Basically she wasn't a just and fair person like Julia. All Elaine thought about was herself. She didn't see how I'd made it possible for her to be a job-share Secretary for years by carrying her (all the other Secretaries didn't know how we managed to make job-share work – the simple answer to that was by me bending over backwards!) It is funny but at the time I couldn't really see this (Julia could!) but only as I look back older and wiser have I realised that there are people in this world who are givers and people who are takers!

I really enjoyed work and my new role. I just kept out of Helen's way. I was always pleasant to her but I just didn't have a lot to do with her. My new job also meant that I didn't have to spend any time working in her office.

Darlington Borough Council at this time was getting ready to become a Unitary Authority. Basically this meant that instead of just being in control of some services and Durham County Council the others, it would have complete control over everything. Everyone knew when it eventually came into place there would be some major changes.

POLES APART

Weeks went by and summer neared its end. I wasn't feeling as happy and in control of things as I had been. Some things began to be an effort. But I just kept plodding on – secure in the knowledge that after all the changes I had made in my life that I couldn't get ill again.

The night before Sue got married me and some of her sisters stayed at her house. We had wine and a girly night. When I later went to bed I lay awake for a while thinking I feel a bit down. I have been looking forward to this wedding for ages and now its here I feel flat.

Sue looked beautiful and radiant on her big day. I was happy for her but although nobody was probably aware of it, I didn't really enjoy myself. Talking to people was a bit of an effort and I wished I could go home early to bed and shut the world out.

About a week or so later I took a Friday off work to sort the house out prior to moving. That evening Julia rang me in a state. Helen had flipped at work and had had a fit on Julia, verbally abusing her. Julia was in shock because two of the girls were witnesses and they didn't go to Julia's aid. Julia just got her bag and said she was going home. She had been crying uncontrollably all afternoon and Eddie couldn't do anything with her. She said she wasn't going back to work. The pressure and the amount of work we were expected to do was also getting to Julia. I started to panic. I knew that without Julia, who I would totally rely on, things at work would be very tough for me.

We moved to our new house the next day which was a Saturday. We were due to go out with friends that evening for a drink and to celebrate. I remember getting ready, not being able to find anything to fit (I had put weight on again – not loads but enough to make my clothes feel uncomfortable) and wishing I didn't have to go. Whilst we were out, I went to the toilets in the pub and had a cry. It may seem silly but even though I knew I was a bit depressed I didn't think I would have another breakdown.

Our department had merged with another department and now we were a really big department. The directors had to apply for their own jobs. Stephen didn't get a new Directorship in the new Authority. I was gutted. Oh no I'll have to learn a new Director's way etc I thought. We were told we'd have to apply for our jobs. Some people would slot into the new structure automatically, some would have to apply for different posts and some would be made redundant. All this happening couldn't have come at a worst possible time when I'd just taken out a mortgage based on my salary. Because of the way I was feeling I decided I would apply for a Word Processor Operator positiion to alleviate stress.

POLES APART

The Council had also installed a new computer system. Everyone was trying to grasp how it worked. To a lot of staff it didn't have a great impact at first because they could still do their job. But to the secretaries and typists all their work had to go from programmes designed on Word Processors to the new computer system. Working conditions were horrendous. Worse than they'd ever been.

When I went to work on the Monday we moved offices to the floor above. Apart from the furniture we had to move everything ourselves. You could cut the atmosphere with a knife. Me, Elaine, Helen and Gwen were sharing an office. There was a desk for Julia for when, and if, she came back. When I left the room for anything and came back I could tell they had been talking about me (not Gwen she wasn't two faced).

Ray Julia's boss went out to see Julia at her home. He asked her to come back and Helen would be warned about her behavior.

I booked a couple of day's holiday to sort out my new house. Billy had gone back to work on the taxis until Eddie's contract started. I didn't get much done. My mind was all over the place.

When I returned to work Julia also came back and was willing to give work a go, Ray had said he would be supportive. What a load of rubbish. Julia got no support. All the work was piling up because of the problems with the new computer system. The atmosphere was terrible. Helen wasn't speaking. Ray was supposed to have had a word with her but her attitude hadn't changed. Julia only lasted a couple of days. Then as if things couldn't get any worse the new Director started.

I thought he was quite aloof and I didn't like him. Elaine worked for him for a couple of days. Then it was my turn. I sat in the Secretary's office next to his, I was a wreck. He wanted me to type some letters, I couldn't even do one – I couldn't concentrate. The phone was ringing constantly. My department was now a very large department. Customers were asking questions about subjects I knew nothing about e.g. drains, public highways etc. Typical of Darlington Borough Council we were in a new department but new had received no training to allow us to cope with all the new changes. I don't know how I got through the day. I cried all the way home. I collapsed into Billy's arms "Don't worry love we'll get through this – I won't let anything happen to you".

Billy rang Dad and told him I was in a bit of a state. Dad said he'd come and see me next day. I slept fitfully that night but when I woke I had a feeling of dread about me. I went food shopping and when I returned Dad was at home. We had a cuddle. "Don't let them do what they did to you before Shell" said Dad. Little did he know that everything that was happening was totally out of my control?

I went to bed that night and sleep didn't come. I became hysterical. I was jumping around the bed sobbing "Billy, Billy I can't be getting ill again it's not possible, haven't I suffered enough already, is my life going to always be like this?" He held me while I cried my heart out. He hadn't any experience of mental health so he felt at a loss for what to do or say. He just kept saying he would look after me and never leave me.

After a sleepless night for both of us Billy made us some breakfast. We'd been invited to Sunday lunch at our friends, Dave and Carole. Billy thought I wouldn't want to go. I said I'd go. I thought a few drinks and a relaxing atmosphere might do me good.

We went and I tried my best to enjoy myself but I was worried sick. All the old feelings were returning and I was terrified of being that ill again.

Sleep eluded me that night as well. Billy rang the Town Hall and said I was ill next morning.

Billy took a couple of days off to look after me. Each day with no sleep I was sinking deeper and deeper into the abyss. I remember not being aware of anyone or anything – I was in hell! Billy was looking after me and cooking my meals. My appetite had gone again. I struggled to eat anything.

Billy had to go back to work as we needed the money. Mum was going to come round late morning and sit with me. I know if Billy had realised how seriously ill I was he would never have left me for one moment. He would have said "sod the money – what's money!" But of course he just thought I was depressed and needed a rest.

When he left the house something inside me snapped. I needed to get out of the house. I took my dogs to the park. We still had darling Roxy but we also had a lurcher pup called Tess. She was about one by then. I adored my dogs and they loved me. It was a cold winter's day and I remember standing on the big park field. There was nobody about. I became hysterical and starting looking up at the sky and shouting "God, why do you hate me so much, what have I done to deserve this? Haven't I suffered enough? I'm sick of picking myself up and trying. I haven't got any more strength" I wanted to go to heaven and see my Nanna. I was totally psychotic by now and all sorts of irrational thoughts were jumbled up in my mind. Oh no I thought this time I'll end up in Winterton and I'll never get out – no I'd rather be dead. I got the dogs and ran home as fast as my legs could carry me. I left the dogs downstairs and flew upstairs to our bedroom. I threw myself on the bed and (this is going to sound totally crazy but its true) thought I'll stay here in this bed and chew myself to death. I started screaming hysterically, punching myself. It was almost like I was having a fit. This went on for about an hour and I was exhausted when I had finished. I got under the covers. Something sort of "popped" inside me and I got a strange taste in my mouth. I realise now it was adrenaline. My body felt really weird.

Mum arrived and I pretended that I was asleep. When Billy came in from work he looked in on me. I pretended I was asleep. Dr Young did a house call that teatime as she was totally concerned as she was aware of my past history. She came into our bedroom and I thought she'd see I was dying. Of course she saw nothing of the sort. It was as if history was repeating itself. At the depths of my madness I had wanted to escape, get out of the hell that was my mind. But I didn't really want to die. I loved Billy and my family so much. I was just exhausted with no sleep, numb and not thinking about anything but the hell I was in. I was convinced next morning I would be in heaven with my Nanna.

I would say I was in a psychotic state for about three to four days. I wasn't sleeping and hardly eating. My body ached all over and I was convinced it was eating away at itself. Not long now I thought.

Somewhere towards the end of the second week of being off work Billy took me out for a ride in his taxi to get some fresh air. We went to Richmond, a small market town near Darlington. As we went over the bumps on the road my body was in agony. We had a little wander around the shops. Billy got some steaks to cook us a nice tea. He was being so loving but I was numb and dead inside.

When we returned home he suggested I have a nice bath and he would make the meal. Before I went upstairs to have my bath (he ran it for me) he said something that actually registered with me. "I don't care if you never go back to work again, we'll manage and when you're feeling a bit better I'll take you up to Scotland" he said. I was in shock. I lay in the bath, deeply depressed but aware of what I'd done.

Like I have said before, I am writing this book 20 years from the date of my first breakdown and can remember everything, but when I was ill my mind would block out the past and I didn't realise I was falling into the same pit as last time i.e. I was convinced I was dying etc – when I look back I can't believe some of the things I thought but as God is my witness it is all true and shows to fellow sufferers how ill I was. I was desperately sad that I wouldn't see Billy, Mum, Dad or Stu when I died, sad that never again would I sit on the banks of Loch Lomand and drink in their beauty and countless other things I would miss by dying. But the die was cast I couldn't change anything.

We had our tea and I picked at the meal. It was dark outside and Billy was watching TV. Roxy and Tess were cuddled up to him on the couch. I said I was going to the corner shop and did he want anything. He seemed really pleased that I was making an effort. He said he would have a couple of cans of lager and gave me some money. I looked at Billy and the dogs all snug on the couch and left the house. I walked past the shop and just kept walking. I kept to the back alleys so no-one could see me. I didn't know what I was going to do, only that I wasn't going to end up in a mental hospital. It was freezing cold and my hands and feet were numb. It seemed like forever but I had only been missing for a couple of hours. I decided I wanted to see Billy and my "girls" one more time. When I got back home Billy was beside himself with worry. He had stayed at home in case I came back and my brother Stuart had been desperately searching the streets for me. They were overjoyed that I had returned and I was safe and sound. I felt nothing – I was numb!

We went to bed not long after that. I could tell by Billy's regular breathing that he had fallen asleep. I felt like I was hallucinating. I wasn't aware of anything in the room but my mind was spinning round and round. I was sure I could see a face where the light bulb would have been. I was convinced it was my Nanna telling me to end things and she would be waiting for me, she was saying I had suffered enough.

Next day Billy said he'd go to work for a couple of hours but he'd be home by lunchtime. I watched him leave feeling desperately sad but still numb. I went upstairs and threw some clothes on. I gave the dogs a cuddle and I left the house. I knew where I was going – the train station!

I walked as quickly as I could. I was aware that if Billy came home he would know I'd gone missing again. Once I reached the station I waited on the platform with all the other commuters. There was a fast train approaching the platform. I didn't hesitate – I walked to the edge of the platform and jumped. As you will see from countless references I have made about God I am quite religious. But it was what happened next that has made me totally believe. When I jumped it was like invisible hands grasped me and lifted me up. I hit the train (there were witnesses to clarify this) and sort of went into it. The best way I can describe it is like in a cartoon when a character charges into something and then just pops out again unhurt. Then everything went black. The next thing I was aware of was being in the pitch black with something dripping on my face (it was engine diesel) and I could hear a loud tannoy announcing something. Then it came back to me what I'd done. I could feel the tracks under me and I knew I was under the train.

POLES APART

I knew I couldn't possibly be alive so I thought I must be dead and this was my penance. I'm not going to Nanna my soul has got to stay on this track for all eternity I thought.

I don't know how long I lay there for but I became aware of voices and a shaft of light. The voices told me to keep still and they would get me out. I realised I wasn't dead but knew I would definitely end up in Winterton now. I just shut my eyes and pretended I was incoherent. I don't know how they got me out from under that train. I only know it was a miracle. About seven years later a very good friend of mine called Lisa was a student nurse. She was working with some paramedics. They were talking about some of the sights they had seen over the years. One of the paramedics said he would never forget being called to Darlington station as a girl had jumped in front of a train. As witnesses had said it had hit me they knew I'd be dead or severely injured (I ended up needing a couple of stitches on the back of my head). They couldn't believe it when they found me and I was all in one piece and alive. In all their years on the job all the "jumpers" (a term used for people who commit suicide by train) they had had to deal with had all been dead when they arrived. Lisa told them she knew me and I had had a breakdown and was fine now.

As they were getting me out from under the train I blacked out and I can't remember anything else until I came round in the Accident and Emergency

Department of Darlington Memorial Hospital. Everything I have said in this book is the truth and straight from my heart. That's why what I say next will shock some people (probably only people who haven't had mental health problems). I was aware that I should have been dead and thought that God wanted me to suffer for everything I had put everybody through so I would have a slow and painful death in a Mental Institution weeks down the line. I knew that my insides were all chewed up and irreparable. I never thought for one moment at that stage that I had been given a second chance and I was fit and healthy, only mentally ill. As I have said countless times when you are this ill you think all sorts of crazy thoughts.

I will say the nurses at Darlington Memorial Hospital were nice to me and eventually they established who I was. They went to contact my family. I dreaded seeing them. Why do I have to suffer like this I asked myself? I know I am dying why it couldn't have been all over on the tracks. Why do I have to suffer all the interrogations and then still die anyway? My life is over but I'm still suffering.

After a short while Billy arrived. He was in a state and I could tell he'd been crying. He was overjoyed to see me alive and in one piece. His first words were "I love you so much, you're never going back to all that stress at the Town Hall, and we'll sell up and go and live up at Loch Lowman in a caravan. I don't care where we live as long as you are ok. You are bound to get better with all the peace and quiet up there". Somewhere from deep inside me his words registered and I desperately wished this to be true. That I wasn't dying and could go and live up in Loch Lowman away from all the stress and bad memories that Darlington held. Billy didn't know what was going on in my mind so he was just glad I was alive and he was looking to the future.

I couldn't face seeing my Dad but Billy went to see Mum, Dad and Stu first. He told them I was dreading to see them and they had to be gentle with me. They were also just so pleased I was alive.

Eventually I got put on a ward. Not in the psychiatric ward as there were no beds but on a geriatric ward. Billy and my family stayed with me all day. Mum fussed about getting me things to eat etc. even though I couldn't eat. When they all went home that night I looked at all the old people on the ward and thought I'll never know what it feels like to be old.

Some time later that evening I saw a phyciatrist for about ten minutes. I can't remember what he said. On the next day Billy visited me on the afternoons visiting session. Mum and Dad came to the evening session. When Dad saw me in bed surrounded by old people he said "She'll never get better in here". He asked to see which phyciatrist was on duty and Dad said he and Mum would look after me and take me to their house. They agreed to let me go (when I look back you would think I would have been sectioned under the Mental Health Act but I wasn't). They got a taxi and took me back to their house. I had a hot drink and asked to go to bed. I lay in my old bed in my old bedroom and I felt so full of bitterness. Last time I lad laid in this bed was the night before my wedding when I had been so overcome with happiness and hope for the future. Why had it come to this again? Why was I constantly being punished? I had picked myself up from the gutter last time and thought I'd gone far but I was back in the gutter again. I wished God would just put me out of my misery and end it for me.

I heard voices downstairs and recognized Sue's voice and her husband Kev. Why can't I be like Sue I asked myself? She's so strong and this wouldn't happen to her (as I have said previously when you are mentally ill you think you are worthless and everyone has more talent than you).

Sue and Kev left me a card and a present and left. Mum and Dad explained I wouldn't want to see anyone yet. Next morning when I heard Dad leave for work I went into Mum's bedroom and asked if I could have a cuddle. I got into the bed and she hugged me so tightly. It felt nice and how I wished I was a little girl again.

POLES APART

Later that morning Dr. Young came out to visit me. She took Mum to one side and told her she was sending me to Winterton. Mum was horrified. "No we'll look after her" Mum said. Dr. Young said "Michelle is a very, very ill young lady and she needs constant 24 hour care, you can't keep your eyes on her every minute of the day".

So the secret fear that had knawed away at me for ten years was becoming a reality. I was ending up in the loony bin.

Billy and Mum accompanied me in the ambulance to Winterton. I can't remember the journey I just tried to block everything out and pretend it wasn't happening.

What I do remember though is arriving and looking up at this horrible old, decrepit Victorian building, which had in the past been used as a lunatic asylum, and fear clutched at my heart. How was I going to cope?

For the next four weeks this was going to be my home and even after the hell I had been through in the past, nothing could have prepared me for this. This was sheer undiluted hell on earth.

It is a scandal really how in this day and age when there is so much money about and some people think nothing of spending hundreds of pounds on a designer handbag that the most vulnerable, old and weak members of society are easily discarded and forgotten.   Winterton was the NHS at its worst.   It wanted knocking down and rebuilding. The rooms and corridors stank of old age and decay.   It wasn't bright and cheerful.   The whole colour scheme was depressing.   I remember clearly when Angie came to visit me she said "How is anyone supposed to get better in this depressing hellhole?"

I got two bunches of flowers and the staff struggled to find two vases to put them in.   There should have been flowers around to cheer people up.   When visitors came at designated visiting times there was one tiny visiting room.   The furniture was old and smelly and there wasn't room to swing a cat.   That was the only room available.   You couldn't talk in private to your loved ones.

When I arrived on that first day Billy wanted to take me straight home but he couldn't – I was sectioned by then. I was in such shock I couldn't even cry I was numb. I was shown where I would sleep in a communal ward with other woman patients. Mum and Billy stayed a short while then they were told they had to go. Billy had voiced his fears that I was very vulnerable and soft-hearted. "There will be nobody violent near her will they?" said Billy. Billy was told that all the really violent patients were in another wing. In my wing there were serious mental health patients like me i.e. Manic Depressives, schizophrenics, drug addicts, alcoholics and people with senile dementia.

POLES APART

I wanted to go to bed to hide but I wasn't allowed. All your human rights are taken from you. You are told when to go to bed, when to eat and when to sleep. You couldn't go and have a nap in the middle of the day if you fancied it.

The food was terrible. It seemed to me as just because we were mentally ill any old crap would do. Some of the nursing staff were ok, some couldn't have cared a less – it was just a job to them.

My ward consisted of a communal day room that held a TV in it with chairs around the TV. There were some tables and chairs for eating on, reading etc. A kitchen, some bathrooms, a couple of consulting rooms, a visiting room and the dormitory style wards.

On my first night I had no choice but to sit in the communal day room. I sat in front of the TV. There was an old man in a wheelchair. He had a male nurse beside him. The old man stared at me and started to bang his leg on the side of the wheelchair and say "Blondie, Blondie, and Blondie" over and over again (I had blonde hair). He was leering at me. I was so uncomfortable but the nurse didn't bat an eyelid. Clearly the old man had senile dementia but nobody cared how vulnerable I felt.

I went to the toilet accompanied by a nurse. I wasn't allowed anywhere on my own that first night (I was on suicide watch). I nearly fainted. As I was clearly in a state they let me go to bed a bit early. My bed was next to the nurse's station. I was allowed no curtains around me for privacy. All night the lights from their office glared into my eyes. Nothing could have prepared me for when the patients arrived to go to bed. Some of them sounded as hard as nails – I lay in bed terrified. When the noise calmed down, one of them started walking up and down the middle of the ward pretending she was Princess Dianna. She was saying "No Charles you can't f**k me!"

I didn't sleep. I lay awake all night. Every hour or so the nurses would come in and shine a light in your face to see if you were still alive and hadn't tried to top yourself. There were bars on the windows and the outside lights shone in. It seemed like an eternity but morning eventually came round. At 7 a.m. the nurses barged in shouting that everyone had to get up. They got really stroppy with the ones that wanted a lie-in – you had to get up you didn't have a choice.

The day went by in a blur but something does stand out in my memory. I had put a big thick jumper on that morning and on the afternoon was feeling really hot and bothered. I went to the ward to get changed. I sat on my bed and pulled the curtain around me. I was sat in my trousers and bra and I was just about to pull the new thinner top over my head when the curtains were yanked open and a boy stood there grinning. I was terrified. He didn't do anything he just looked at my breasts and walked out of the ward. Male patients were not supposed to go anywhere near the female ward. I was shaking but decided not to say anything for fear of reprisals. Some of the patients looked and acted like real hard cases. Some of them were drug addicts and not to be messed with. An example of this was when it was meal times you had to stand in a queue. The hard faced ones pushed their way to the front of the queue and had first choice of the food. The weaker and vulnerable just got what was left. One evening I didn't get a hot meal I got a sandwich as that's all there was left.

The days drifted by. The only way I coped was to block everything out. Actually by now I wasn't psychotic (I was on medication by then) just deeply, deeply depressed (dead inside). I didn't make any friends and just kept myself to myself. I didn't trust anybody. Most of them were ill just like me but I wasn't mentally strong enough to put my trust in strangers. I was hardly eating and Billy was really worried about me.

One day Sue and Kev came to visit me. I could tell by their faces they were shocked at the change in me. I didn't say much to them but as they were leaving I took Sue to one side. "Sue you've got to believe me, I didn't want to die under the train, but I was dying anyway, my insides are rotting away. I can taste the poison rotting them". (I still used to have a funny taste in my mouth). Of course Sue knew I was desperately ill and just thought it was the illness talking – which it was.

I saw the resident phyciatrist a few times but he was as mad as a hatter. He used to stalk around Winterton wearing a bowler hat! Some people think that you have to be a bit mad yourself to deal with the mentally ill and I think this is true.

The days blurred into weeks and eventually they said I could go home. Billy had left his job and said he would be my carer. I was pleased to leave Winterton but I could find no joy as I knew I was still dying.

I was let out just before Christmas. I hated every minute of that Christmas. Other people were laughing and merry and me in the pits of hell.

Stuart my brother took me home from Winterton (we didn't have a car) and I was pleased to see Roxy and Tess, my girls. They were overjoyed to see me. Billy said they had been pining a bit. They would sit by the front door and listen for my footsteps. Whilst I was working I always wore heels of some description and they would make a clattering noise. When I would approach the front door on my way home from work they would recognise it as me and get overjoyed at the thought of seeing me.

POLES APART

Even though it was the day before Christmas Eve and early morning (about 10 o'clock) I asked to go to bed. Billy agreed and the dogs followed me upstairs. Billy turned a blind eye. He knew they would be getting on the bed with me. When I was well he would always moan if I had let the dogs on the bed and say it was unhygienic. Poor Billy had other things on his mind besides dog hairs!

Later that day Billy asked if I fancied a bit of fresh air and said we would also get some Christmas presents. I was filled with horror. "Oh no I can't leave the house". He didn't push me. Everybody told Billy not to worry about presents and just look after me. He was brilliant with me but the walls I had put around me in Winterton were still there and I wasn't letting no-one in.

On Christmas Day at Mum's house, Mum got me a cross-stitch kit. I just looked at it and thought I'll never do that. But later that day when they all went to the pub for a couple of drinks, Billy had fallen asleep, I couldn't watch TV, I picked up the tapestry. It was quite complicated but I persevered. Whilst I was doing the tapestry I didn't think about my problems and enjoyed doing it. For the next couple of years cross-stitch became a life-line for me. They became something else to focus on besides myself.

Weeks turned into months and time dragged by. It was my second breakdown all over again with my thinking, daily, hourly of what I'd miss when I was dead. Billy did all the shopping and cooking. Occasionally I would go to the supermarket with him but this terrified me so much I tried to avoid going. We never socialized as a couple anymore. But I would stay at Mum and Dad's one night a week (usually a Sunday) and Billy could get a break and a night out. The only people I ever saw were Billy and my family. I saw Sue and Angie occasionally but I didn't want contact with other people.

My good friend Lisa (whose house we had bought) lived in a bigger house down the street. She had just given birth to twins before my breakdown and she would call regularly but I wasn't often up to seeing her. Her life seemed so perfect that when she left I would be eaten up with jealousy. In my deeply depressed eyes everything good just seemed to land in her lap. (She had a baby, Sean, when she was 17 but her husband Simon (then her boyfriend) had a well paid job. She lived in a lovely house, didn't have to go out to work, drove a nice car, had regular holidays abroad, went out socializing a lot, no money worries and to top it all had just had two gorgeous twin girls). I only had all these feelings while I was ill, Lisa turned out to be a good friend while I was ill and was always ringing or calling and enquiring how I was or could she help in any way.

Because I didn't think I had a future my mind would go over and over the past. How I'd always tried my best but people would walk all over me.

POLES APART

I'd always been a giver and not a taker but look how I'd ended up. I'd always given work 100% but they couldn't have cared a less about me. There were no caring sympathetic letters enquiring about my welfare. I got a bunch of flowers and a card from the staff in my department when I was in Winterton but that was a long time ago. When I used to worry about work Dad used to say to me "Shell that place will still be standing when you are ten feet under". He was saying everyone is just a number, easily replaced and just as easily forgotten. To this day I have never received a leaving present or card. I was there for eleven years and I know I was well liked and respected at my job but I had committed the crime of being mentally ill – the last taboo! I was just that sad, silly Michelle with everything going for her who threw it all away in their eyes.

Julia was still on the sick from work also. She was deeply depressed. She had had a breakdown also. She had never suffered with her nerves in her life until she went to the Town Hall. We talked occasionally but we were both too ill to really help each other.

A lady called Sue from the Union came to see me, she was very understanding. She had seen my case against the Council when I had my second breakdown so she totally understood what had happened.

After a time Julia did go back to work but not to the Town Hall. By then the new unitary Council was so big it had to acquire additional office space. So Julia wasn't working at the Town Hall in the centre of town, she was working in council offices in a different part of the town. Also she was working with different people. She said it was hard but she was taking it day-by-day. I was pleased for her but knew I'd never work again.

One day when she'd been at work a while she rang me. She was a lot stronger by then. Julia said me and her should make a joint claim against the Council for the stress they had put us under with no backing from management. I didn't have the strength to be knocked back again. Anyway what was the point, by the time, if and when, it went to Court, I would be dead anyway.

Sue from the Union came out to see me again (I'd been on the sick for over a year). She asked if I would consider going back to work in another department or building. I don't know to this day why I agreed to give it a try.

She sorted it out for me to work in Economic Development, a small section of the new department I was in. It was housed in a separate building in the town centre fairly near the Town Hall. I was to be a Word Processor Operator with the chance (if I wanted to) of being a secretary to the manager there eventually.

POLES APART

Billy put no pressure on me but I seem to remember Dad thinking it was a good idea to give work one last chance. (It is only in the last few years that I have totally come to realise all my breakdowns were work related – Dad didn't realise they were solely work related or he would have said never go back). At twenty eight I was a bit young to be on the scrap heap work wise. I just went along with it.

I got myself in a state the night before I was due to start. I even lay in bed plotting how I could get out of it. For a split second I even thought about trying to get hit by a car as we crossed the road but knew that wouldn't be fair to Billy or the driver.

I hated every second of being back at work. I was only working a couple of hours a day. The staff in my new section were fairly nice to me but I felt awkward and like a fish out of water. I was still no where near my old confident self (how could I be when I was still convinced that I was dying). I lasted about three days. On about the fourth day I became hysterical when it came to the time for Billy to take me to work. He calmed me down and said I didn't have to do anything I didn't want to do. He contacted Sue from the Union. She came to see me. I told her I was never going back to the Council again. She set the ball in motion and eventually I got medically retired. I didn't even get a pension as I had opted out of the council's scheme years prior (bad pension advice by a Financial Advisor). I got three months wages and that was it? The hatred I felt towards the Council knew no bounds.

Now ten years later I think I have had the last laugh. When I was ill I couldn't go past the building. If I was in a car or taxi and could see it in the distance I would shake with fear. But now I swan past and feel like sticking my two fingers up at all the backstabbers all hard away working and I think of my lovely life now, with Billy and my angels, Kristy and Lauren, that I have had to fight tooth and nail to get.

We bought a car with my severance pay. Billy started taking me out for day trips. Looking back there are lots of similarities from my second breakdown. During the day when we were doing things I tried to focus on what we were doing and enjoy it. It was only at night that the negative fears of dying etc came into my mind. I even had a couple of nights out at our local pub with Billy. The first time was horrendous, as although most of the people were nice, they were at a loss as how to treat me and I felt awkward. Although we only went out drinking occasionally, each time got slightly better.

It is funny when I look back and think my second breakdown happened five years before my third and I can remember things more clearly. Nothing in particular stands out with my third. Time just plodded on. I didn't go wandering on my own any more. Because I was free now from the one big controlling force in my life – THE TOWN HALL – I did start to feel a bit like my old self. This made me sad because I knew if I hadn't decided to chew myself to death on the bed that day I would be well and happy and looking to the future. Even though I was definitely improving there was a small part of me that would see no reason – I was dying and that was a fact. Mum, Dad and Billy didn't know I felt like this. Some days when we had a nice day out, we would return home and because the fear of dying and leaving Billy would become too much, I would break down crying in front of Billy. "Billy, Billy I'm scared of dying and going to hell" I would say "Don't Shell" he would say "You're scaring me". He thought I was going to try and top myself again. I just kept my thoughts and fears to myself and plodded on. I saw a Phyciatrist once in a blue moon and they were hopeless.

One day Sue came to see me and tell me that she had some news. She was pregnant. I was pleased for her – if anybody deserved this Sue did – but I couldn't help think I'll never hold a baby in my arms that belongs to me.

We were invited to a friend of Billy's little boys christening. I spent days before hand doing a cross stitch as a present and didn't mind going. Most of the people there had seen me since I became ill so I wasn't that apprehensive.

It was quite a nice day. The party afterwards took place at Chris and Dianne's house (the parents). The party was in full swing when I began to feel unwell. I felt like I was coming down with a cold and I also felt sick. Billy took me home and put me to bed. After a couple of days of being poorly in bed and feeling no better Billy made an appointment at the Doctors for me. When I saw Doctor Young she checked me over and asked me to do a pregnancy test. I thought this was a total waste of time. How could I be pregnant? I was dying, my insides were irreparable.

She told me to ring up for my results in a week's time. I never gave it much thought. I knew I wasn't pregnant. I did ring for my results and when she said it was positive I was shocked for a moment. Then the negative side of my brain took over. Your body's just tricking you – you can't possibly be pregnant.

Billy, my family and friends were all pleased. They all thought a baby would give me something to focus on. If I hadn't had my secret fears I would have agreed wholeheartedly. Although I was always into my career, I have a strong maternal instinct and I love to mother things. As I have said before, I treat my dogs like babies. I was very secretive throughout my "pregnancy". When the midwife came out to fill in all the paperwork and check me over, I was supposed to ring the hospital to fix up a date for my scan. I "lost" the letter. As luck, or unluck, would have it, I slipped through the net and it wasn't until I was about five and a half months pregnant that the midwife realised I hadn't had a scan. I didn't want a scan as I knew there would be no baby only my ill dying body. I knew they'd take me back into hospital and I would never get out until I died. I would rather spend what little time I had left with Billy. When the Gynecologist saw I had never had a scan I said I did not want one now as if there was something wrong with the baby I did not want to know – I would not have an abortion I told them. I only said all this so they would think I was not ill anymore and coping with my pregnancy.

The crazy thing is I had all the symptoms of being pregnant. I had terrible morning sickness. My "bump" grew but I was on another planet.

I kept up the pretence with everybody. Sue is the only person I have ever told about how I felt during the whole of my pregnancy. I didn't tell her at the time only years later. When it was near my time I got a second hand pram and kept it at Mams. What was the point in getting a new one – no baby would be using it. About a month before the baby was due Billy decorated one of the spare rooms as a nursery. Mum and Dad had got me some essentials i.e. mosses basket, changing table, blankets, nappies etc. When he had finished the room Billy popped out to the shops for something. I sat in the new nursery and broke my heart. How I desperately wished I was having a baby and it would sleep in this lovely room. How happy I would be.

My due date came and went. I had to go to see the Gynecologist. I was huge by now. Prior to getting pregnant I was all skin and bone (Billy was always worrying about my weight before I got pregnant as I hardly ate anything). I had put on about four stone. He said if the baby had not made an appearance by Sunday – it was a Wednesday when I went to see him – they would "start me off".

That night I sat on the toilet and cried as if my heart was breaking. I knew the end was near. Once they got me in hospital and saw inside me via scans etc. they would see what I saw and that would be it. These would be my last few days with Billy. Of course Billy just thought I was overcome with emotion because the baby had not come yet and I was worried, tired etc. He cuddled me and said "Don't worry it will be fine".

I went to bed early and hardly slept. Next morning I was getting ready to go to Mums. I had been to the toilet. I was walking down the stairs when some water started trickling down my leg – it felt weird. When I saw Mum I told her. She said "I think your waters have broken". She rang the hospital. They told her to bring me in. Billy and Mum accompanied me to the hospital. I was petrified. Here it was the day I had dreaded had come round.

POLES APART

I was in "labour" all day. From early evening to about ten pm they said I was making good progress, 'then nothing'. The "baby" was getting stuck in the birth canal. I was on gas and air and not thinking about anything. In the early hours of the morning they said I had to have an emergency caesarean. I signed a form but was too weary to comprehend what was going on. I remember them getting me ready for surgery. The anesthetist put a needle in my arm, 'then blackness'.

The next thing I remember is Billy's face smiling down on me. "Well done Shell darling we have got a lovely little girl" – he gently placed this little bundle in my arms – my baby!

I spent the day in complete shock. How could I have a baby? All my family and friends were overjoyed. There was a constant stream of visitors. I was in a side ward all of my own. When everybody had gone home at the end of the evening visiting session there was just me and Kristy (Billy loved that name – he's Scottish). What happened in the next few minutes were going to alter the course of the rest of our lives? My precious baby and me. I I picked her up out of her cot and cuddled her into me. I went to sit in a chair by the window. It was dark outside but I looked up into the dark sky and focused on a star. Everything seemed to become clearer as if the mist was clearing out of my head. I couldn't be dying. How could a dying body give birth to a healthy child? Even if I did die one or two years down the line, I was going to live each day to the full and give thanks for my precious gift.

I was true to my word and that was the day I moved forward. I loved being a mother and took to it like a duck to water. I went a bit high as I was overcome with happiness but leveled off again.

I enjoyed motherhood so much that sixteen months later our darling Lauren came into the world. My life was complete. I was not afraid of the future anymore. I had two precious lives to fight for. Even if I did become ill again I would get help straight away. I would walk over molten coals to protect and keep my children happy. After all children are one of life's precious free gifts – the best gift of all!

CONCLUSION

It has been a total soul searching experience writing this book. I have had to delve so far back in the past and dig up memories and things that happened that I thought I had forgotten. But never underestimate the capacity of the human mind - it stores everything and never forgets!

Every fact is true but some small minor details I may have got mixed up i.e. dates as I have gone back as far as twenty years.

POLES APART

It has been very therapeutic for me. I have cried many tears whilst writing it, but also smiled with joy. Because if you have come this far you will see my life so far has been a rollercoaster of very highs and very, very lows.

Although I have been both happy and "depressed" in the last twenty years I feel I have been in a wilderness struggling to find out who I am. Now I finally know who I am. Some people will say I have changed. No this is the real me – the one that got "lost". [I am what I am and what I am needs no excuses, life's not worth a dam till you can shout out I AM WHAT I AM – quote from Gloria Gaynor's famous song. If people don't like me well that's their hard luck – Tough! I like me, no I LOVE ME!

There are so many sufferers out there just like me. It is so hard and frustrating when people don't understand. Even my own parents don't understand totally and Dad has had one breakdown. I don't like to criticize my parents because I love them dearly but sometimes I think they think they "got me well". Yes I was lucky they were there for me but surely even with the best parents in the world it has to come from the individual. (You can take a duck to water but you can't make it swim). They understand depression but they don't understand serious mental illness. When I was psychotic I was very ill and all the delusions I had i.e. dying were caused by me being ill.

Some days I feel it is an uphill struggle, but one I am determined to win, not only for my own self worth but for my Nanna's memory. This is mainly caused by other people's negative attitudes and misunderstandings. I am a normal, intelligent and caring individual who has an illness through no fault of mine. Only about three times in my life I have lost touch with reality and the rest of the time I am just as astute as anybody else, if not more so than some. I may get a bit hyper but I am still sane, so please don't patronize me, or people like me, as if we are idiots and play mind games with us. A couple of acquaintances of mine pussyfoot around me and sometimes say hurtful things. But if I respond back they turn it round and say it's all in my mind. This is so frustrating. For years I have chewed myself when things like this happen but since I started writing everything down I have become stronger. I now think I am the better person. I would never treat anyone like that [do unto others as you would have you] they are just ignorant and cruel. You should never look down on someone and judge them too harshly. For I believe "what comes around goes around". The people who laugh and scoff at mental illness may find themselves ill one day!

Blame is a strong word and whilst I don't blame anybody for what happened to me, Darlington Borough Council, and in particular, the men who were paid very well to manage me, failed me appallingly. They could never have predicted my first breakdown and when I was ill at seventeen, Brian Cook, the Office Manager, was very supportive. He would ring my parents to enquire after me and this was a major factor in me getting well. That I felt I had support at work. But they could have stopped my second and third breakdowns. I left Darlington Borough Council ten years ago, I have given birth to my two darling angels, Kirsty and Lauren within sixteen months of each other, had money worries, Billy has been made redundant more than one, suffered bereavement when my lovely Nanna died (dad's Mum) and yet I have never had another breakdown.

The Town Hall was the major cause of my breakdowns and through them I could have been dead, my husband and my family's lives ruined. They would have said "She was a nice girl Michelle but what a stupid thing to do". Never would they have attached any blame to themselves and by now I would be a long forgotten memory.

I know for some reason I wasn't meant to die. I would like to believe that I've been given this second chance to help others. Many people may scoff at this and think it is a bit far fetched but whilst writing this book I was also reading a book which was number one of the New York Times Best Seller List entitled "Chicken Soup for the Woman's Soul". It is full of true stories to make you think and rekindle your spirit. One particular chapter is headed "Live Your Dream". My dream, which I hope to achieve, is to become a Motivational Speaker on bi-polar and stress at work. I am not looking for material gain but if by telling my story and speaking to people I could motivate someone to seek help and change the course of their life for the better my Nanna's life won't have been in vain.

I dedicate this book to you Nanna!

With all my love, and fondest memories.

I hope and prey to see you when my time comes in the ever lasting valley of peace and love.

Michelle, xxxxx

www.ingramcontent.com/pod-product-compliance
Lightning Source LLC
Chambersburg PA
CBHW031209270326
41931CB00006B/480